PUBLIC POLICY AND THE DENTAL CARE MARKET

Evaluative Studies

This series of studies seeks to bring about greater understanding and promote continuing review of the activities and functions of the federal government. Each study focuses on a specific program, evaluating its costs and efficiency, the extent to which it achieves its objectives, and the major alternative means—public and private—for reaching those objectives. Yale Brozen, professor of economics at the University of Chicago and an adjunct scholar of the American Enterprise Institute for Public Policy Research, is the director of the program.

PUBLIC POLICY AND THE DENTAL CARE MARKET

Alex R. Maurizi

American Enterprise Institute for Public Policy Research
Washington, D. C.

This study is one of a series published by the American Enterprise Institute as part of the research program of AEI's Center for Health Policy Research. A distinguished advisory committee, whose members are listed below, helps guide this program.

The director of the Center for Health Policy Research is Robert B. Helms.

ISBN 0-8447-3189-7

Evaluative Studies 24, November 1975

Library of Congress Catalog Card No. 75-34646

Printed in the United States of America

CONTENTS

	INTRODUCTION		1
I	A LEGISLATIVE SUMMARY		3
	Government Action: the Supply Side	3	
	Government Action: the Demand Side	6	
	Outline of the Study	8	
II	EVALUATION OF THE SUPPLY PROGRAMS		9
	The Decision to Enter Dentistry	9	
	An Evaluation of the Scholarship Program	14	
	An Evaluation of the Dental School Construction Program	18	
	Summary	20	
III	THE IMPACT OF NATIONAL DENTAL HEALTH INSURANCE PROGRAMS		23
	Dental Services: Demand and Supply	23	
	Model Estimation	24	
	Using the Model for Policy Analysis	25	
	Summary	29	
IV	AN EVALUATION OF THE REGULATORY POLICIES		31
	Regulatory Functions	31	
	The Data Used in the Analysis	32	
	Measuring the Impact of the Regulations	33	
	Summary	37	
V	THE RATIONALE FOR GOVERNMENT INTERVENTION		39
	Externalities or Neighborhood Effects	39	
	Imperfect Capital Markets	41	

Imperfect Information ... 44
Income Redistribution ... 44
Summary ... 46

VI **SUMMARY AND CONCLUSIONS** ... **49**

APPENDIX A: Specifications of the Various HPEA Loan, Scholarship, Construction and Formula Grant Expenditures ... **53**

APPENDIX B: Rates of Return and Dental Enrollments ... **57**

APPENDIX C: The Two-Stage Estimation Procedure Used in the Two-Equation Model in Chapter 3 ... **61**

APPENDIX D: The Impact of the Regulations on the Earnings of Dentists ... **65**

NOTES ... **67**

TABLES

1. Federal Funds for All Health Manpower Programs, by Type of Support, Selected Periods, 1957-1972 ... 4
2. Federal Funds to Dental Schools and Students under the Health Professions Educational Assistance Programs, 1965-1972 ... 5
3. Vacancies in the Freshman Class, All U.S. Dental Schools (and Puerto Rico), 1959-1971 ... 12
4. Basic Data on Dental Enrollments, Applicants and Rates of Return, Selected Years ... 13
5. Dental Rates of Return, Assuming Existing Tuition and Full-Cost Tuition, Selected Years, 1948-1970 ... 19
6. Predicted Number of Applicants to Dental School, Assuming Existing Tuition and Full-Cost Tuition, Selected Years, 1948-1970 ... 21
7. Means and Standard Deviations for 1961, and Elasticities of Variables Appearing in the Model ... 25
8. Equilibrium Values of Dental Prices and Quantities: Different Insurance Programs and Policy Options ... 27
9. Amount and Source of Loan Funds for Dental Students, by Source ... 43

B-1 Testing for Possible Autocorrelation ... 58

INTRODUCTION

The large-scale entrance of the federal government into the dental care market began with the Health Professions Educational Assistance Act of 1963 and the development of the Medicaid program for the poor in 1965. The 1963 act and subsequent legislation involved the federal government on the supply side, whereas Medicaid brought federal involvement on the demand side. Today, interest in a universal, national dental insurance program is increasing. If such a program were enacted, it would greatly step up the government's role on the demand side of the dental care market.

This study evaluates the effectiveness of some of the programs on the supply side and estimates the probable impact a national dental insurance program would have on the dental care market. In addition, it examines some of the regulatory policies followed at the state level. Their relation to national policy needs more careful consideration than it has been given in the past.

Chapter 1 provides a brief history of legislation affecting the dental care market between 1963 and 1974. Chapter 2 evaluates the federal dental student scholarship program and the federal dental school construction program. Chapter 3 considers the probable impact of national dental insurance on dental prices and the quantity of dental services and looks at other federal policies that might be pursued in conjunction with a national dental insurance program. Chapter 4 looks at the impact of the powers of dental licensing boards on the earnings of dentists. Chapter 5 examines the rationale for federal intervention in the dental care market, suggesting which programs appear to be appropriate and which do not.

CHAPTER I

A LEGISLATIVE SUMMARY

Public action in the dental care market has taken several forms. On the demand side, the principal development in the last decade has been federal and state financing of the purchase of dental care among the nation's poor through Medicaid. Current discussion of a national dental insurance program at the federal level proposes extending this policy to all citizens. On the supply side, the principal development in the last decade has been the federal subsidy of dental school construction and of dental students through the Health Professions Educational Assistance Act. At the state level public policy has continued its past role in the regulatory arena. Both federal and state public action are discussed in detail below.

Government Action: the Supply Side

The Health Professions Educational Assistance Act of 1963 (HPEA, Public Law 88–129) and its subsequent modifications were designed to avoid what was described as a looming critical shortage of medical personnel.[1] Total expenditures for health manpower programs over the period from 1965 to 1972 are summarized in Table 1 according to the type of assistance provided; total expenditures for these programs over the period from 1957 to 1964 are also presented for purposes of comparison. Over 89 percent of all expenditures over the period from 1957 through 1972 were made in the period from 1965 through 1972. Table 2 presents total expenditures for dentistry for each year according to the category of assistance.

The objective of the federal program for dentistry was to increase the number of dental personnel so that the 1975 practitioner-to-population ratio would be the same as the 1962 practitioner-to-

Table 1

FEDERAL FUNDS FOR ALL HEALTH MANPOWER PROGRAMS, BY TYPE OF SUPPORT, SELECTED PERIODS, 1957–1972

($ thousands)

	Period		
Support Category	1957–1964	1965–1972	Total 1957–1972
All categories	$305,777	$2,490,893	$2,796,670
Construction growth	276,180	1,116,827	1,393,007
Formula grants	7,423	473,534	480,957
Special project grants	7,412	325,975	333,387
Student loans	0	282,256	282,256
Scholarships	0	124,463	124,463
Traineeships	14,762	149,029	163,791

Source: Bureau of Health Manpower Education, *Trends in Program Statistics: Grants, Awards, and Loans, FY 1957–1972* (Washington, D. C.: U.S. Department of Health, Education and Welfare, 1973), p. 5.

population ratio. It had been estimated that without a federal program, there would be a shortage amounting to 12,000 dentists by 1975. In order to avoid this shortage, it had been estimated that the number of dental school graduates would have to increase from 3,000 per year in 1962 to 6,200 by 1975. The fifty-four schools existing in 1962 would need to expand by about 750 places, and twenty-two new schools, each graduating 100 dentists per year, would need to be built. Such large increases in enrollment and in capacity, it was thought, could be accomplished only with federal help.[2]

Student Support. The passage of the HPEA established both a loan program and a scholarship program for medical personnel. Of the approximately $361 million of federal HPEA funds spent for dentistry over the period from 1965 to 1972, approximately $44 million went for loans and $14 million for scholarships. (Nursing, medicine and dentistry received the bulk of all expenditures among all categories from 1965 through 1972. Nursing, medicine and dentistry received 38 percent, 36 percent and 16 percent of all loan expenditures, respectively; and they received 44 percent, 27 percent and 11 percent of all scholarship expenditures, respectively.)[3] Since the programs were begun there has been considerable variation in the

Table 2

FEDERAL FUNDS TO DENTAL SCHOOLS AND STUDENTS UNDER THE HEALTH PROFESSIONS EDUCATIONAL ASSISTANCE PROGRAMS, 1965–1972

($ thousands)

	Year								
Support Category	1965	1966	1967	1968	1969	1970	1971	1972	Total 1965–1972
School construction	$19,180	$14,997	$35,539	$23,521	$24,108	$29,642	$25,787	$ 1,268	$174,042
Institutional support									
Formula support		2,975	8,441	8,862	9,213	9,204	9,120	34,988	82,803
Special project support		0	0	2,689	8,723	12,962	15,845	6,773	46,992
Student support									
Loans	2,871	4,624	7,132	6,822	6,778	3,584	5,471	6,636	43,918
Scholarships			808	1,476	2,354	3,165	3,005	2,893	13,701
Total									361,456

Source: Bureau of Health Manpower Education, *Trends in Program Statistics: Grants, Awards, and Loans, FY 1957–1972* (Washington, D. C.: U.S. Department of Health, Education and Welfare, 1973), pp. 6, 13, 35, 45, 61, 65.

interest rates charged on the loans, in the maximum loan or scholarship amount, in eligibility requirements and in loan repayment terms. The reader is referred to Appendix A for a discussion of these changes.

Dental School Support. Support for dental schools took two principal forms under the 1963 act and subsequent amendments. First, construction grants-in-aid were provided for new teaching facilities and to replace or rehabilitate existing teaching facilities. The new facilities constructed could be either new schools or additions to existing schools. Second, a basic program of institutional support was provided. This program consisted of a formula grant based on the number of students and graduates. Bonuses were given for enrollment increases beyond a mandatory increase required to qualify for support. Dental school construction grants amounted to $174 million from 1965 through 1972, while formula grant expenditures amounted to almost $83 million. These two programs combined accounted for over 70 percent of the $361 million in federal expenditures on dental manpower programs: the details are presented in Table 2.

Government Action: the Demand Side

The participation of federal and state governments in financing the purchase of dental care has been slight in comparison with their participation in financing the purchase of medical care. The two major programs currently in operation, Medicare for the elderly and Medicaid for the poor (enacted in 1965 as Title 18 and Title 14, respectively, of the amendments to the Social Security Act), expended a total of approximately $22 billion in 1974.[4] Medicare expenditures are made primarily for physician and hospital expenses and are almost entirely federally financed. Medicaid expenditures, on the other hand, can be made at the option of the states, for such things as dental care, optometric care, and nursing care. Medicaid is financed jointly by the federal and state governments, with the federal share ranging from 50 percent to 85 percent.[5]

The rapid rise in Medicaid expenditures, from less than $2.0 billion in 1966 to over $8.0 billion in 1972, occasioned considerable criticism of the program.[6] Expenditures for dental care under Medicaid, which averaged 3.1 percent of the total in 1970, have also risen rapidly if we are to judge by evidence from the states of California, Massachusetts, and New York.[7]

One recent study found that increases in Medicaid costs have come primarily from increases in the number of persons eligible;

rising prices and participation rates have been contributing factors.[8] Obviously, any national dental insurance program is likely to have a significant impact on total expenditures for dental care. Chapter 3 provides an analysis of the impact of a dental insurance program on total dental expenditures.

Regulatory Policy. Public policy at the state level affects the dental care market on both the supply and demand sides through the regulatory functions of the states. The history of legislation in this area will not be described here since it is otherwise available to the interested reader.[9] A brief summary of the major features of this regulatory policy, however, is given below.

To practice dentistry, one must obtain a license from the state in which the practice is to be located. The requirements for licensure are usually determined by a state dental licensing board or a state dental practice act. To apply for a license, an applicant generally must have graduated from an accredited school of dentistry and be a U.S. citizen. Accreditation of schools, the length of dental training required, the requirements for admission to dental school, and the dental school curriculum are determined on the basis of rules adopted by the House of Delegates of the American Dental Association and in accord with the policy established by the Council on Dental Education of the American Dental Association. The nature of the examination to be taken for licensure is determined by the state dental licensing board. There is a national theoretical examination now accepted by most state licensing boards, but until the recent development of regional boards every state had its own clinical examination. Few states have reciprocal arrangements to allow a practicing dentist to relocate without taking the license exam in the state where he relocates.

Once the dentist is allowed to begin practice in a state, the nature of his practice is determined by the practice regulations in that state. These regulations generally define the procedures and practices reserved for the dentist alone and the behavior allowed the dental firm. For example, the duties performed by the dental hygienist or dental assistant generally exclude the drilling and filling of cavities and the administering of anesthetics.

Although licensing was originally intended to protect the public from dishonest and incompetent practitioners, increased attention has been given to the possibility that licensing powers are not being used in the public interest.[10] By the imposition of unnecessarily difficult requirements for obtaining a license, the number of practitioners may be kept lower and their earnings kept higher than would otherwise be the case. Since all members of most dental licensing boards are required to be dentists, and since many state dental associations have been established for the purpose of promoting dental licensing legislation and have helped select the members of state dental licensing boards, there clearly exists an opportunity for members of a state's dental profession to use the licensing power in their own interest. Evidence suggests that the members of some licensed occupations do derive benefits from the use of their licensing powers in the form of higher prices for their services.[11]

In addition to these effects on the supply side, regulations at the state level affect the demand side by altering patterns of consumer search behavior. Since dentists are usually not allowed to advertise their location, the kind of services offered, or the price of services offered, consumer search is more costly than it would be if advertising were permitted.

Chapter 4 provides an analysis of the impact of two important supply-side aspects of dental licensure on the earnings of dentists. This analysis is used to assess the extent to which dental licensing boards use their power in a manner inconsistent with the public interest.

Outline of the Study

This study examines each of the elements of public intervention in the dental care market. It attempts to assess and evaluate their impact on the dental care market, and concludes that the public policy actions on the supply side have been expensive and inefficient, as well as concluding that the development of a universal national dental insurance program is likely to be quite expensive. Finally, it concludes that state regulatory actions have reduced the earnings of dentists (and thus the return on their education) in some states and have increased their earnings (and thus the return on their education) in other states.

CHAPTER II

EVALUATION OF THE SUPPLY PROGRAMS

The largest supply-side expenditure program provides dental school construction grants. One of the smaller programs provides dental student scholarships. Both are evaluated here with the aid of a model of human investment behavior applied to the behavior of a student considering dentistry as a professional career.

The Decision to Enter Dentistry

The training necessary to be a dentist may be thought of as an investment in human capital.[1] This investment yields a lifetime income stream, namely the excess of the lifetime earnings of a dentist over the earnings that would be obtained without this dental training. The cost of dental training (that is, the investment) consists of the direct costs incurred during training along with the income foregone during training as a result of the decision to become a dentist. Since the decision to enter dental school is made after two, three, or four years of college, the income stream foregone is that of the second-, third-, or fourth-year college student. Direct costs during training consist of tuition costs, supply and equipment costs, and the cost of books. Of course, while in training, the dental student earns income during the school year and during summers, and his wife (if he is married) may be willing to work in order to help him through school. These additional earnings are all counted on the return side of the investment, along with whatever scholarship aid the student receives. The expected return on this investment is defined either to be the present value of the returns minus the present value of the costs or to be the rate of return which is similar to the rate of profit earned by a firm from its investment.[2]

Of course, the dental student may be influenced in his decision by a number of non-monetary factors. Dentistry offers an opportunity for the exercise of mechanical skills just as medicine does. In contrast to medicine, however, dentistry involves shorter and more regular hours with few occasions for emergency calls at odd hours of the night or on weekends. The opportunity to be of service to his fellow human beings and the professional status which dentistry provides are likely to be important if not paramount considerations to the prospective dental student. To suggest that the decision to enter dentistry is to be viewed as an investment in human capital is not to suggest that these other considerations are unimportant,[3] but rather that their importance changes slowly over time in comparison to the financial returns on the investment so that behavior may be reliably predicted by examining the returns on investment in dental training. Of course, there are information and decision lags in dentistry, just as there are in other fields such as engineering,[4] so it is likely that the changes in the financial attractiveness of dentistry relative to the financial attractiveness of alternative professions will have a lagged effect on the decision to enter dental school. The lag may be even more pronounced for dentistry than for (say) engineering, since the college student interested in a dental career is allowed to enroll in dental school after either two, three, or four years of college. The student may have an incentive to remain in college an extra year or two as a hedge and to determine the trend in the financial attractiveness of a dental career.

To make sure this human investment approach to the decision to enter dental school is appropriate, we must demonstrate first that the potential dental student has some idea about his future earnings as a dentist. The evidence available on this point suggests that the potential dental student does have a fairly good idea about his future earnings. Applicants to dental school in 1958, when asked to estimate what their dental earnings would be after five years in practice, came up with an average net-earnings estimate of $11,922.[5] According to the 1959 American Dental Association Survey, the average 1958 net income of all dentists aged thirty to thirty-four amounted to $12,527.[6] Of course, students forming estimates of their future earnings on the basis of available information about dental earnings at a given point in time will tend to underestimate their future earnings the further into the future they look unless they allow for the overall growth in the incomes of dentists and of college graduates,[7] but even so, they may not be underestimating either the real value of the earnings or the differential between earnings as a dentist and earnings in some other profession.

The Theoretical Structure. The supply of labor to a particular occupation will depend upon the financial attractiveness of that occupation relative to the financial attractiveness of alternative occupations.[8] Unfortunately, there are no data on the rate of return for what might be an alternative profession for dental students, such as that of being a physician.[9] (There is indication that many dental students would consider medicine as an alternative; about 90 percent of one sample of Canadian students who were accepted at both a medical and a dental school chose to enroll in a medical school.)[10] We have therefore chosen to examine the impact on supply of the dental rate of return relative to the return on long-term (ten-to-fifteen-year) government securities; the latter is considered to be a proxy for the returns on investment choices other than dentistry.

The supply of labor to any occupation is a *relative* supply, that is, relative to the numbers eligible to enter the occupation. We have attempted to measure the relative supply by using the number of dental enrollments and of dental school applicants divided by the number of eligibles. The number of eligibles is measured by the number of individuals earning bachelor's or first degrees in the physical and biological sciences. Since about 90 percent of all dental school applicants in 1958 majored in biology, chemistry, or premedical science,[11] this measure seems to be a reasonable one. It should be pointed out, however, that only 63 percent of dental students had a bachelor's degree before entering dental school in 1970. This percentage has been increasing steadily over time, growing to 63 percent from 30 percent in 1949.[12] It is likely, though, that the greater the number of earned bachelor's degrees in the physical and biological sciences, the greater will be the number of second- and third-year college students majoring in these fields. In any event, there appears to be no other available measure of the number of individuals who have the interest and skills required for entry to dental school.

The relative rate of return for the calendar year preceding enrollment is expected to influence relative applicants and enrollments in any given year (t). This is apparent from the definition of applicants and enrollments as follows. An applicant to dental school in any given year (t) is defined as a person who took the Dental Admission test in April or October of the preceding year ($t-1$), or January of the given year (t), and requested that the results be sent to a dental school to satisfy one of the requirements for entry in the fall of that year.[13] Thus, a person applying for admission in the fall of 1971, for example, would be taking the admission test in April 1970, October 1970, or January 1971. For most students the decision to apply for admission in the fall of 1971 is expected to be influenced by the rate of return on investment in 1970. The applicants in 1971 would be drawn from a pool of eligibles graduating in June 1971. The relative rate of return in calendar year 1970 is thus expected to influence the number of 1971 applicants relative to 1971 graduates. New enrollments are assumed to be a subset of applicants in the same year and, hence, are also expected to be influenced by the rate of return in the preceding year ($t-1$). Since students may apply for admission in one year, be denied, and apply again in the next year or year after, and since students may apply and be accepted in one year and decide not to enroll until the next year or year after, relative enrollments expected to be influenced by relative rates of return in year t are averaged over the years $t+1$ to $t+3$.

Finally, enrollments are limited to the number of dental school places. Since vacancy data collected since 1959 (displayed in Table 3) indicate that enrollments have been at or near capacity, enrollment

Table 3

VACANCIES IN THE FRESHMAN CLASS, ALL U.S. DENTAL SCHOOLS (AND PUERTO RICO), 1959–1971

Year	Vacancies (percent)	Enrollment	Capacity
1959	3.8	3,607	3,748
1960	4.3	3,648	3,812
1961	4.0	3,646	3,999
1962	3.7	3,680	3,820
1963	1.2	3,770	3,813
1964	.1	3,836	3,839
1965	1.0	3,806	3,842
1966	2.1	3,942	4,025
1967	.8	4,200	4,233
1968	.5	4,203	4,221
1969	—[a]	4,355	—[a]
1970	—[a]	4,565	—[a]
1971	1.6	4,745	4,822

[a] Note should be made that, according to Thomas Ginley, capacity data and vacancy rates for these years were not calculated since it was widely believed that vacancy rates were zero or close to zero, and capacity therefore the same as enrollments.

Source: Thomas Ginley, Council on Dental Education, American Dental Association.

changes may be no more than a reflection of capacity changes which may, in turn, be determined by exogenous factors. To the extent that more students would have enrolled had there been places for them, enrollments cannot be used to determine the ability of financial returns to provide our society with its supply of dentists. Applicant behavior, however, is not as likely to be similarly affected by capacity constraints and can be used to better determine whether there is a need for subsidies.

The Empirical Results. The data utilized in the analysis are presented in Table 4. The regression analysis is presented in Appendix B. The results are statistically significant (see Appendix B for more detail). The rate-of-return elasticity evaluated at the point of means is .69 for enrollments and .76 for applicants. This means that a 10 percent increase in the return to dental training relative to the interest rate on U.S. government securities increases relative dental

Table 4

BASIC DATA ON DENTAL ENROLLMENTS, APPLICANTS AND RATES OF RETURN, SELECTED YEARS

Year	(1) Dental Rate of Return $(R)_t$	(2) Interest Rate $(i)_t$	(3) Freshman Enroll-ments (average) $\overline{E}$	(4) Applicants $(A)_{t+1}$	(5) Pool of Eligibles (average) $\overline{B}$	(6) Pool of Eligibles $(B)_{t+1}$
1948	17.6	2.4	3,180	8,407[a]	26,070	24,921
1952	19.0	2.7	3,349	5,178	19,644	20,121
1955	16.4	2.8	3,589	7,376	26,600	24,238
1958	13.6	3.4	3,598	6,498	31,326	30,609
1961	15.3	3.9	3,762	6,566	36,252	32,908
1964	21.7	4.2	3,982	9,988	44,747	43,220
1967	21.1	4.8	4,374	9,037	55,959	51,497
1970	25.5	6.6	5,176	11,012	57,390	57,155

[a] Applicants in 1949 are approximated by one-half the sum of 1948 and 1950 applicants since 1949 applicant data are unavailable.

Sources: Column (1): Maurizi, *Economic Essays,* p. 13; more recent data calculated by the author. Column (2): Council of Economic Advisers, *Economic Report of the President, 1973,* p. 260. Column (3): Council on Dental Education, *Dental Student Register, Annual Report,* annual. Column (4): Council on Dental Education, American Dental Association. Columns (5) and (6): Bureau of the Census, *U.S. Statistical Abstract,* "Earned Degrees Conferred by Field of Study & Level of Degree," annual.

enrollments by 7 percent and relative dental applicants by almost 8 percent. These results can be used to assess the impact and cost of the dental scholarship aid program and the dental school construction program.

An Evaluation of the Scholarship Program

As of 1960, less than 2 percent of all dental students received scholarship aid.[14] As a result of the scholarship program, the proportion of dental students who received scholarship aid increased to 5.3 percent in 1967 (the first year scholarship funds were disbursed to dental students) and to 24.7 percent in 1970. The average amount of per capita aid received was $1,012 in 1967 and $773 in 1970.[15] The expected annual scholarship assistance thus amounted to $54 (1012 x .053) in 1967 and $191 (773 x .247) in 1970. The effect of this aid (with nothing else taken into account) was to increase the rate of return to dentistry from 21.0 to 21.1 percent in 1967 and from 25.1 to 25.5 percent in 1970.

There were considerable variations in the criteria according to which the dental schools disbursed the scholarship funds intended to help students with exceptional financial needs. Ideally, if scholarship administrators had perfect knowledge of each person's financial situation, the aid would go only to individuals who would not attend dental school otherwise. In the absence of this perfect knowledge, it would be expected that the aid would go only to those students with the fewest financial resources and whose parents had the lowest income and fewest assets. However, a recent examination of the scholarship program indicates that scholarships were not awarded to students on criteria that were uniform throughout the dental schools and were not even awarded to students considered to have the greatest need according to a given school's own criteria.[16] In addition, scholarship aid awarded to needy students often far exceeded their needs.[17] Consequently, it seems reasonable to suppose that the typical dental student had a chance of obtaining aid whether or not he was in need of it. In the absence of a better estimate, we shall consider the percentage of students receiving aid in 1970 (24.7) multiplied by the average amount of aid received in 1970 ($773) to estimate the amount of aid the typical student would expect to receive. The effect of this aid on enrollments may then be computed using equation (1) of Appendix B; the effect on applicants may be computed using equation (2) of Appendix B.

Equation (1) of Appendix B predicts that a rate of return of 25.5 percent would generate an average enrollment level in the

1971–73 period of 5,335 students. This amounts to 53 more than the enrollment level of 5,282 predicted assuming a 25.1 percent rate of return. Equation (2) of Appendix B predicts that a 25.5 percent return would result in 11,044 applicants in 1970, or 122 more than the 10,922 applicants predicted assuming a 25.1 percent return.

The data in Table 2 indicate that $3.165 million was disbursed in scholarship aid in 1970. An enrollment increase resulting from this aid amounting to only 53 students means that it cost approximately $59,716 for every additional student permanently enrolled for four years. The annual cost for each additional student enrolled amounts to $14,929. This is far greater than the average amount of $773 of aid per student and the figure would suggest that only one out of every nineteen students receiving aid actually decided to enroll because of it. In other words, there was a substantial amount of leakage in the scholarship program. Most of the students receiving aid would have attended dental school anyway. Even if all of the additional 122 applicants had been able to enroll, the per student cost would still have amounted to $25,943 or $6,486 annually. In this case, only one out of every eight students receiving aid would have enrolled because of it.

The reasons for this leakage are not hard to find: they reside for the most part in the administration of the aid program. The schools have not been adequately instructed on how to distinguish cases of exceptional financial need (which are eligible for scholarship aid) from cases of financial need (which are eligible for loans). As a result, there has been considerable variation in the methods the schools have used to determine exceptional need; these methods were often inconsistent or unrelated to the intent of the legislation. Specifically, the schools had to decide the amount of the student's resources, whether the student was self-supporting, the amount of expenses to be allowed, and the type of expenses to be allowed.[18]

The Determination of the Student's Financial Resources. Only 75 percent of the schools involved subscribed to the College Scholarship Service, which measures a family's financial resources and anticipated educational expenses and determines the amount of support that a student's parents can contribute to his educational expenses, in order to determine the student's need.[19] The remaining schools have used their own system to determine the amount of parental support. As a result, one student attending a school in the former group (the group using the service) and coming from a family of two children, whose family income totalled $11,000 and whose family assets totalled $25,400, was considered able to obtain $1,580 from his parents while one student attending a school in the latter group (the group not using the service), also coming from a family of two children, whose family income was $11,150, and whose family's assets were $27,000 was considered able to obtain only $770 from his parents.[20]

Even among schools using the College Scholarship Service, some disregard the figure or adjust it in some way. In one case, the aid officer in the school adjusted the figure at his discretion but did not document the basis for the adjustment.[21] In another case, the computed parental contribution of $2,500 was reduced to $1,300 by the aid officer because the student's parents had another child attending college, despite the fact that the College Scholarship Service had adjusted its computations to account for the second child attending college.[22]

Determining Self-Supporting Status. There has been considerable variation among the schools in the way in which it is determined whether a student is self-supporting. Some schools defined all students under twenty-five years old to be dependent unless it could be demonstrated that the student did not receive parental support and was not being claimed as a dependent for tax purposes.[23] Some schools defined a student as self-supporting upon receipt of a notarized affidavit of nonsupport from the parents.[24] Some schools defined these as independent but also included veterans and those married for more than two years or having children.[25] Some schools made subjective decisions in each case.[26] The variation in results may be indicated by the following examples.

In one case—this one related to a student at a medical school—such a self-supporting student's parents had an income of $24,500 and assets of $26,000; the parents were determined to be able to contribute $6,000 to the student's education. Yet, since the student declared himself self-supporting, his parents' financial situation was disregarded in determining his need.[27] In another similar case, a self-supporting medical student received a $2,100 loan and a $900 scholarship. Yet the student's parents had an $11,000 income and assets of over $100,000 of which $23,000 was in cash.[28] In still another case, a self-supporting medical student received a $1,600 loan and an $800 scholarship. He was twenty-six years old, married, and had two children; his parents had an income of $31,000 and owned assets totalling $820,000 in value. The College Scholarship Service calculated that his parents were able to contribute over $12,000 toward his educational expenses which the school estimated at $6,700.[29]

Determination of Student Expenses. In trying to determine the expenses involved in attending school, 75 percent of the schools developed standard budgets; the remainder used expenses estimated by the student in his application to determine the expenses involved in his attending school.[30] As a result, there was aid provided for legitimate items but in excessive amounts and also aid provided for questionable expenses. Some dental student budgets included such items as books, equipment, and supplies for amounts ranging from $300 to $1,500 more than the actual cost.[31] Other student budgets included such expenses as $850 a year for clothing, laundry, and cleaning, $390 a year for toiletries and personal grooming, $225 a month for automobile maintenance and transportation, and $360 a month for housing.[32] One dental student was allowed a budget of $11,119 which included—in addition to expenses for tuition, books, instruments, food, lodging, clothing, and travel—$250 for personal expenses, $301 for insurance, $1,740 for miscellaneous expenditures, and $2,208 for automobile operation.[33] Another dental student was allowed a budget of $13,191 which included $6,532 for unexplained miscellaneous expenses.[34]

Variation in the Amount of Aid Received. As these examples demonstrate, there has indeed been considerable variation in the amount of aid awarded and in its relation to need. Dental students in one school's freshman class all received $200 in scholarship aid, yet their needs, as defined by the College Scholarship Service, ranged from zero to over $8,000.[35] In another school, one student whose costs amounted to S6,900 and whose resources were estimated at $500 received a scholarship of $1,450 while another student who indicated costs of $6,400 and resources amounting to $11,600 received a scholarship of $2,500.[36] Nor is this the end of the story, for in addition to obtaining aid under HPEA, a number of students were able to obtain aid from other federal sources. Several examples will serve to illustrate.

One student received a $900 loan and $300 scholarship under HPEA and also obtained $2,760 in veterans educational assistance benefits, and a $2,000 insured loan, a $1,353 tuition payment, and a $2,773 stipend payment under the Uniformed Services Health Professions Revitalization Act (USHPRA) which was provided by the Navy. This student's need was computed to be $2,965.[37]

Another student received a $1,000 loan and a $600 scholarship under HPEA, a $3,207 state fellowship, and $6,279 from the Navy under USHPRA. His needs were computed to be $4,080.[38]

Nor are these isolated examples. One school estimated that two-thirds of all the students receiving aid under HPEA were also receiving aid other than from HPEA.[39]

Had the administrators of the scholarship program been able to identify those students who attended dental school only because of the scholarship aid they were able to obtain and provide such aid to these persons alone, the money would have been used most efficiently and the cost of each additional student enrolled would have been the amount of aid he received. However, since the administrators of the program provided aid to many students who were not in need and who would probably have attended dental school even without the aid, the cost of each additional student enrolled by the program has been extremely high.

Undoubtedly, one reason for this high cost is the fact that the schools have administered the program with inadequate guidelines. Another reason is that it is a scholarship program rather than a program providing loans at or near market rates of interest. When individuals are required to repay the aid they receive, they are much more likely to take the aid only if they believe it is worth their while to borrow the money and later repay it. They are likely to spend the borrowed money more wisely than they would spend outright grants.

Considering the current high rate of return being earned by dental students on their training, it is difficult to understand why a government loan program at market rates of interest would not be sufficient to guarantee a supply of dental personnel. (Indeed, as will be discussed later, it is even questionable whether a government loan program to dental students is really necessary in view of the fact that the typical dental student is considered a good credit risk by private lending institutions.) That the Congress has considered phasing out the scholarship program may indicate some realization of this.

An Evaluation of the Dental School Construction Program

The rationale underlying the construction subsidies to dental schools must be that there would be inadequate incentive for the dental schools to expand without the construction subsidy. This is somewhat difficult to understand in view of the fact that dentistry would be a profitable investment for most dental students even if they were required to pay the full costs of their education.

Since the dental student on average pays about one-third of the full cost of his dental education,[40] equations (1) and (2) of Appendix B can be used to estimate the impact of full-cost tuition on applicants and enrollments by supposing tuition to be triple what it was in each of the years observed. Table 5 presents rates of return calculated under the assumption of full-cost tuition payments alongside rates calculated assuming one-third of full-cost tuition. The percentage drop in the rate of return varies from 17 to 30 percent and averages 21 percent over the entire period.

Assuming full-cost tuition, enrollment would nevertheless have increased from a predicted average level of 4,362 students in 1965–1967 to 4,604 students in 1971–1973, an increase of 242 students. Under the same assumption, applicants would have increased from a level of 8,817 in 1964 to 9,373 in 1970, an increase of 556 applicants. The number of additional freshman dental school places constructed using the construction subsidy funds amounted to 1,123 between 1965 and 1971.[42] Thus, had students been paying full-cost tuition, enrollment would have increased by 242 students, so the cost of the construction subsidy should be calculated on the difference between 1,123 and 242, or 881 students. The $174 million spent by the federal government between 1965 and 1971 for the construction of added dental school places really generated 881 places. The federal cost per place would then amount to at least $197,503 instead of the $154,942 calculated by assuming none of the 1,123 added places would have been generated in the absence of the construction subsidy.

If, in addition to assuming full-cost tuition we assume that a completely unsubsidized private-dental-school market were to pre-

Table 5

DENTAL RATES OF RETURN, ASSUMING EXISTING TUITION AND FULL-COST TUITION, SELECTED YEARS, 1948–1970

	Rate of Return	
Year	Existing tuition	Full-cost tuition
1948	17.6	13.5
1952	19.0	15.0
1955	16.4	11.4
1958	13.6	11.3
1961	15.3	12.3
1964	21.7	17.5
1967	21.1	17.1
1970	25.5	19.9

Source: Data in Table 4, and equations in Appendix B.

vail with unrestricted entry (that is, no approval or accreditation required), then we could reasonably expect that enrollments would have at least increased from the number of applicants predicted in 1964 assuming full-cost tuition (8,817), to the number of applicants predicted in 1970 assuming full-cost tuition (9,373). This increase (556 students) would mean that of the 1,123 places added, only 567 would have been generated by the construction subsidy. The federal cost per place would then amount to $306,878.

Of course, it should be pointed out that so large a change in the nature of the dental school market would have further ramifications that a statistical estimate based on the previous historical record might not be able to capture. Dental schools would be more likely, in such a completely new setting, to find more efficient ways to instruct their students and use their faculty members or physical plant. There would likely be substantial reductions in the length of the training period, achieved by shortening the length of courses or discarding courses wherever possible. Such changes as these would increase dentistry's financial attractiveness and would likely lead to further increases in the number of applicants and enrollments. Thus, our estimate of the extent of enrollment increase in an unsubsidized private market may be too low, and our estimate of the federal cost per dental school place constructed, though it may appear high, may still be too low.

It should be pointed out that average enrollment levels fell short of predicted applicant levels over the entire period under study. Table 6 presents the relevant data for this comparison. The comparison indicates that, even if we assume full-cost tuition, the predicted number of applicants ran between 1.34 and 2.21 times the average enrollment levels over the period. That is, on the average, a completely private unsubsidized competitive dental school market could have provided our society with at least 75 percent more freshman dental students than have been provided by the existing arrangement. With full-cost tuition, dental schools might have increased capacity more rapidly than they did with government subsidy and they would not have lacked applicants to fill the larger number of places made available.

Summary

The federal government has subsidized the supply of dentists by providing loans and scholarships to students, assisting in the construction of additional dental school places, and providing funds to the dental schools for additional enrollments and special projects.

Table 6

PREDICTED NUMBER OF APPLICANTS TO DENTAL SCHOOL, ASSUMING EXISTING TUITION AND FULL-COST TUITION, SELECTED YEARS, 1948–1970

Year t	Average Freshman Enrollments $t+1$ to $t+3$	Predicted Applicants, Year $t+1$ — Linear Form	
		Existing tuition	Full-cost tuition
1948	3,180	7,837	6,355
1952	3,349	6,120	5,070
1955	3,589	6,367	4,848
1958	3,598	6,060	5,326
1961	3,762	6,423	5,528
1964	3,982	10,321	8,817
1967	4,374	10,917	9,424
1970	5,176	11,036	9,373

Source: Data in Table 4, equations in Appendix B.

An evaluation of the student scholarship and school construction programs indicates that these programs have been extraordinarily expensive and have provided only modest results. They may even have been counterproductive. Only a small fraction of students receiving scholarships would have decided not to enroll in dental school in the absence of a scholarship program, and many of the dental school places constructed with federal funds would have been built anyway in an unsubsidized dental school market. The sizable amount of wasted resources resulting from these two programs calls their need into question, especially in view of the rate of return being earned by the average dental student on his investment in dental training.

This chapter did not evaluate the federal loan program to dental students. A discussion of the rationale for such a program is presented in Chapter 5.

CHAPTER III

THE IMPACT OF NATIONAL DENTAL HEALTH INSURANCE PROGRAMS

As was noted earlier, dental insurance programs are simply transfers of income from the general taxpaying population to the recipients for the purpose of providing for their purchase of additional dental care. The costly Medicaid experience makes it imperative for us to estimate the impact a large-scale transfer program would have on the dental care market. In order to determine what the impact of such a program would be on the price of dental care, on the quantity of dental services, on the total expenditure on dental care and on the overall federal expenditure on dental care, it will be necessary for us to develop a simple model of the demand for dental services and the supply of dental services.[1]

It is important to note at the outset that this model measures the demand for and supply of dental services. It is not a model of the demand for and supply of dentists, although the quantity of dental services and the quantity of dentists are obviously related to each other. Concentration on dental services will allow us to examine the effects of such things as changes in the number of auxiliaries upon the supply of dental services and, therefore, will enable us to examine the impact of policy decisions affecting the number of auxiliaries.

Dental Services: Demand and Supply

Demand. The demand for dental services is affected by a number of factors.[2] Here we assume demand to be a function of the price of dental services, the income level of consumers, and the extent of fluoridation. The higher the price of a dental visit, the fewer the number of dental visits that will be demanded. The income level of consumers and the extent of fluoridation are considered to be parameters which affect the location of the demand curve. The higher consumer incomes are, the greater the amount of dental services consumers will want to buy at each possible price. An increase in incomes thus shifts the demand curve outward. The presence of fluoride in the drinking water is expected to reduce the quantity of dental services that people want to buy at each possible price since fluoridation is a dental caries prevention measure. An increase in the extent of fluoridation thus shifts the demand curve inward.[3]

Supply. We consider the supply of dental services to be a function of the price of those services, the number of chairs in the dental office, the number of assistants in the dental office, and the number of hours worked by the dentist in his office.[4] The supply of dental services is also, of course, affected by such factors as the extent of technical change in the industry. Technical advances in drilling equipment, particularly the development of high-speed drills of between 30,000 and 100,000 RPM and of those in excess of 100,000 RPM,[5] have made it possible for dentists to treat more patients in a given time period. One estimate puts the increase in productivity from high-speed drilling equipment at about 1.2 percent per year.[6] However, since the data used for estimation did not include information on the speed of the drills used by the dentist, this factor could not be included.[7]

Model Estimation

The results of the two-stage least squares estimation process for this simple two-equation model are displayed in Appendix C. In Table 7 are given the means and standard deviations of each of the variables together with the elasticity (evaluated at the point of means) for the variables in the demand equation and for the price variable in the supply equation.

The data suggest that the demand for patient sittings is quite elastic with respect to price; the value of −1.76 is somewhat larger than the −1.43 estimated by Paul Feldstein.[8] The income elasticity of 1.06 is quite similar to the .99 permanent income elasticity observed by Anderson and Benham for dental expenditures, taking into account price, quality, demographic variables and preventive care, but lower than the 1.24 permanent income elasticity they observed when these other variables were not taken into account.[9] It may be noted, however, that some have estimated an income elas-

Table 7

MEANS AND STANDARD DEVIATIONS FOR 1961, AND ELASTICITIES OF VARIABLES APPEARING IN THE MODEL

Variable	Mean	Standard Deviation	Elasticity
Q	3279	1463	
P	12.99	1.95	Supply: .79 Demand: −1.76
PCY	2128	459	1.06
FL	28.5	18.8	−.40
K	2.2	.8	
AX	1.3	.7	
HRS	1963	423	

Note: Q = quantity of dental services
P = price of dental services
PCY = consumer income
FL = extent of fluoridation
K = number of chairs in the office
AX = number of full-time auxiliaries
HRS = number of hours worked annually by the dentist

Source: See Appendix C.

ticity for dental expenditures as high as 2.0.[10] Feldstein estimated the income elasticity at 1.71 in his model.[11] The supply of patient sittings is not as price elastic (elasticity of .79) as is the demand. However, our estimated price elasticity is greater than the .29 estimated by Feldstein.[12]

Using the Model for Policy Analysis

In order for us to determine the impact of a national dental insurance program, it will first be necessary to determine what market prices and quantities would be, in equilibrium, in the absence of such a program. Comparing equilibrium prices and quantities under the program with equilibrium prices and quantities in the absence of the program will provide a means of isolating the impact of the program itself. The determination of equilibrium prices and quantities from our model is explained in Appendix C.[13]

In order for us to determine the actual equilibrium values for P and Q in a specified year, it will be necessary to assign values to all of the exogenous variables. Let us, therefore, determine the equilibrium values of P and Q for the year 1970. Values of PCY, K, AX, and HRS for 1970 and a value of FL for 1969 are assigned:[14] the resulting equilibrium P and Q values are displayed in Table 8 under the heading "no insurance program." The equilibrium price for a patient sitting in 1970 would have been $15.62 and the equilibrium number of sittings would have been 4,476. The gross income of the typical dental practice would have been $69,920. Given 92,984 active, non-federal dentists in 1969,[15] this would imply a total expenditure of $6,501 million.

In order for us to determine what the equilibrium values of P and Q would have been in 1970 with a dental insurance program in effect, let us assume that the program was a simple one in which the federal government paid 80 percent of the price for all dental expenditures of all persons in the country. In other words, let us assume a universal plan with a 20 percent copayment feature—that is, the plan has no deductible feature and the copayment percentage does not vary with income.[16] The price elasticity of demand evaluated at the equilibrium values of $15.62 and 4,476 sittings is −1.56. The percentage increase in the number of sittings demanded with such a plan would, therefore, be (1.56) (80) = 125 percent. In the very short run, immediately after the initiation of such a program, consumers could be expected to respond as though prices had actually fallen by 80 percent. But before the program had been in existence for very long, consumers would discover that their incomes had in effect risen considerably. They would be able to purchase all the dental care they had previously purchased and would also purchase (with the same income) more dental care than they had previously. The effects of the insurance program on prices and quantities can be examined by supposing that consumer incomes for exogenous reasons had risen sufficiently (the demand curve had shifted outward) to cause the same increase in the quantity of sittings demanded.[17] The details for this procedure may be found in Appendix C. This new value for per capita incomes could then be substituted into the reduced form equations (3) and (4) of Appendix C along with all the same values for the other variables in order to determine a new equilibrium P and Q. The results of these calculations appear in Table 8 for a 20 percent copayment and for a 50 percent copayment program. With a 50 percent copayment program, the price per sitting would be $22.07 and the number of sittings would be 5,121 per dentist in the new equilibrium position; with a 20 percent copayment program, the price per sitting would rise to $25.83 and the number of sittings would be 5,497 per dentist. Thus, the program would cause prices to rise by 41 percent with

Table 8

EQUILIBRIUM VALUES OF DENTAL PRICES AND QUANTITIES: DIFFERENT INSURANCE PROGRAMS AND POLICY OPTIONS

	Policy Options											
	Auxiliaries not doubled No additional fluoride			Auxiliaries doubled No additional fluoride			Auxiliaries not doubled Fluoride = 60%			Auxiliaries doubled plus fluoride = 60%		
Variable	No Ins.	50% Co-Pay	20% Co-Pay	No Ins.	50% Co-Pay	20% Co-Pay	No Ins.	50% Co-Pay	20% Co-Pay	No Ins.	50% Co-Pay	20% Co-Pay
Equilibrium Price	$15.62	$22.07	$25.83	$14.03	$19.76	$23.21	$14.48	$21.56	$25.12	$12.89	$18.12	$21.32
Equilibrium Quantity	4,476	5,121	5,497	5,186	5,760	6,742	4,398	4,992	5,348	5,108	5,631	5,951
Total Expenditures[a]	$6,501	$10,509	$13,202	$6,765	$10,583	$14,550	$5,922	$10,008	$12,491	$6,122	$9,487	$11,798
Total Federal Expenditures[a]		$5,254	$10,502		$5,292	$11,640		$5,004	$9,993		$4,743	$9,438

[a] In millions.

Source: See text and Appendix C.

50 percent copayment and by 65 percent with 20 percent copayment, while the number of sittings would rise by 14 percent in the first instance and 23 percent in the second instance. These results reflect the fact that the demand for sittings is much more price-elastic than is the supply of sittings. Total expenditures would rise by 62 percent in the first instance (to $10,509 million) and by 103 percent in the second instance (to $13,202 million). Total federal expenditures would be $5,254 million annually in the first instance and $10,562 million, or 101 percent higher, in the second instance.

The model may be used to assess the effects of other policy variables. Let us suppose, for example, that the state laws preventing the delegating of additional tasks to the dentists' auxiliaries were relaxed, and let us suppose the effect of having an expanded duty auxiliary instead of the traditional auxiliary is the same as the effect of having two traditional auxiliaries. If we double the number of auxiliaries from 1.56 to 3.12 in our model, the effect will be to lower prices and substantially increase the quantity of sittings, as Table 8 shows. The addition of an insurance program under these conditions would mean that total expenditures would be only slightly greater, at $10,583 million, as against $10,509 million assuming 50 percent copayment or at $14,550 million as against $13,202 million assuming 20 percent copayment. Total federal expenditures would be correspondingly higher at $5,292 million and $11,640 million (compared to $5,254 million and $10,562 million) annually.

We might also inquire about the impact of increasing the extent of fluoridation, say, from 43 percent to 60 percent. The effect of this change alone would be to decrease prices and to decrease sittings; total expenditures are reduced by almost $600 million annually in the no-insurance case. Total expenditures would be $10,008 million ($500 million less) assuming 50 percent copayment and $12,491 million ($700 million less) assuming 20 percent copayment. Federal expenditures would be $5,004 million and $9,993 million, respectively.

Let us suppose, now, that both these policy actions are taken. The results are given in Table 8. The combined effect would be to decrease prices and increase sittings. Under a 50 percent copayment program, total expenditures would be $9,487 million; the federal share of this would be $4,743 million. Under a 20 percent copayment program, total expenditures would be $11,798 million; the federal share of this would be $9,438 million.

The difference between federal expenditures under a 50 percent copayment and federal expenditures under a 20 percent copayment program remains roughly a factor of two no matter what other policy variables are manipulated. The difference between the most and least expensive policy combination is sizable, however, amounting to over $2 billion annually ($11,640 million as against $9,438 million).

Summary

Using a simple model of the national dental care sector, we have demonstrated that a universal dental insurance program could increase total expenditures to more than twice the level they would be without it, assuming a copayment percentage as low as 20 percent. Federal expenditures would vary not only according to the copayment percentage, of course, but also according to what age and income groups are covered under the program and according to what kinds of treatment are covered under the program. In our model, for the sake of simplicity and in order to isolate the impact of the various policy choices, we have assumed coverage to be universal.

These conclusions are based, not on a forecast of what will happen in the future, but rather on a calculation of what would have happened in the past (1970) if a universal insurance program had been in effect. The information obtained from this exercise can nevertheless guide current policy choices by indicating the relative magnitudes of expenditure involved.

No attempt has been made to estimate the expense involved in providing so-called "free" care—that is, a program in which the federal government pays all dental bills. It seems reasonable to assume that the expense would be at least as great as the expense of a 20 percent copayment program.

CHAPTER IV

AN EVALUATION OF THE REGULATORY POLICIES

In this country the price of dentistry is regulated at the state level. Each state requires that anyone proposing to practice dentistry in the state obtain a license issued by the state. The criteria which must be met by anyone who wishes to obtain a license together with the criteria which must be met by anyone who wishes to keep his license constitute the regulations surrounding the practice of dentistry.

By 1907 all states in this country had established laws which provided for the licensure of dentists.[1] In most cases, these laws were passed as a result of strong support from the dentists in each state, arguing—through their state dental society or association—[2] that the licensure of dentists was required to protect the public interest against unqualified practitioners. It should be noted that dentists do not differ substantially from the other health professionals who are licensed in states throughout the country. The principal question concerning licensure, for dentistry or any other profession, is whether the public interest has really been protected. Some economic theorists suggest that licensing laws are established solely to promote the interests of the profession or occupation seeking licensure.[3] The fact that licensing is sought by the profession rather than by its clients, it is argued, substantiates this view. Although we cannot fully resolve this issue here, we can indicate whether the dental licensing laws have indeed served the interest of dentists.

Regulatory Functions

The licensing law provisions grant the authority to determine whether a dental school is to be accredited (graduation from an accredited dental school is generally required for licensure),[4] whether a dental student from an accredited school is allowed to take the licensure examination (U.S. citizenship is generally also required),[5] and whether a person who takes the examination passes or fails it. Also included is the authority to recognize the license of a practicing dentist from another state (the basis of reciprocity agreements among states which allow practicing dentists in some states to relocate freely across some state lines).[6]

The licensing law provisions also grant the authority to determine the organization and functioning of a dental practice by specifying the duties of the dentist and his auxiliaries, if any,[7] and the way in which the dentist conducts his practice. The dentist, in most cases, may not advertise the location of his practice or the fees he charges for his services, for example.[8]

It is not possible for us to examine the impact of every regulation, so we will devote our attention to the impact of the regulations in two important areas: (1) the power to establish a state licensing examination and to determine who shall pass and who shall fail; and (2) the power to allow the expanded use of dental auxiliaries. The impact of the regulations on the financial interests of the dentists in each state is approximated by their effect on the average hourly earnings of all dentists in that state. The contention that the provisions of the licensing laws are designed to promote the financial interests of the dentists will thus be directly evaluated.

In order to conduct this evaluation, it will be necessary for us to examine the earnings of dentists in each state, control for all those factors which we would expect to influence a dentist's earnings, and then examine the impact of the regulatory powers on the dentist's earnings. Unfortunately, only a sample population of dentists is available on which to conduct such an analysis. Moreover, not all the factors which could be expected to influence a dentist's earnings can be controlled for. Nevertheless, some important conclusions can be drawn from such an investigation.

The Data Used in the Analysis

The sample population of dentists used is the 1970 Census Public Use Sample (one-in-one-hundred sample) of dentists in the civilian labor force. Although this sample of dentists is not particularly large (it consists of 858 dentists), it appears to be the only source of disaggregated data on individual dentists available for the recent past.

It should be pointed out that these Census data have several important characteristics which affect our analysis. The Public Use

Sample includes data from both respondents and non-respondents. The information for each person sampled indicates the questions for which the recorded data represent a response from the person sampled and those for which the data represent a non-response whose missing value was then estimated by the Census Bureau.[9] Only those dentists who responded to all the questions relevant to this analysis were included; this limitation had the effect of reducing the initial sample of 858 dentists to 801 dentists.

Second, the Census data do not provide us with direct information on a dentist's earnings per hour. Rather, they provide information on the dentist's earnings during the year 1969, the number of weeks worked during the year 1969, and the number of hours worked during the week of the 1970 Census (in April 1970). Hourly earnings in 1969 must be approximated from this information by dividing 1969 earnings with a product of 1969 weeks worked and 1970 hours worked per week. This estimate is subject to some bias. In particular, serious bias results from the inclusion of recently graduated dentists who did not work or worked part-time until graduation in 1969 and then worked full-time for the remainder of 1969 and through the survey week in April 1970. Reported annual earnings would be too low for 1969 and reported hours worked would be too high for 1969, thus causing the approximation for hourly earnings for this group to be biased downward by a substantial amount. Accordingly, all dentists with one year or less of experience in the labor force (labor force experience is approximated by the difference between age and the summation of the number of years of education plus six) were excluded from the analysis. The number of dentists in this category was approximately 4 percent of the sample. Also, in order to reduce bias in the estimate of hourly earnings, only dentists who worked full-time were included in the analysis, where full-time hours were defined to be working more than thirty-five hours per week in 1970 and also more than forty-five weeks in 1969.

Finally, because of sample size limitations, the analysis was conducted on white male dentists. The result of all the limitations imposed on the sample was to reduce the sample of 858 dentists to a sample of 420 dentists. It is upon this sample of 420 dentists that the analysis was conducted.

Measuring the Impact of the Regulations

As was noted above, only two important regulatory functions will be examined: (1) the function of passing or failing applicants for a state's licensure examination; and (2) the function of allowing expanded-duty auxiliary personnel to be assigned many of the office tasks traditionally performed by the dentist himself.

The ability to control the number of dentists practicing in a state by altering the pass/fail rate should be expected to have an impact on the earnings of dentists in that state.[10] The higher the state's failure rate, over time, the greater the hourly earnings of the dentists in that state can be expected to be.[11] We have, therefore, used the average of the yearly failure rates on the state examination over the period from 1960 through 1969 as a variable which we expect to be positively associated with the hourly earnings of dentists in that state.[12] The higher the failure rate during the decade, the higher the hourly earnings we expect in 1969.

The ability to allow dentists to delegate office tasks should also be expected to have an impact on dental earnings. Although the delegation of office tasks to what are termed "expanded-duty" auxiliaries is a fairly recent phenomenon, there is sufficient information for 1969 on the differences among states in this regard to enable us to examine its impact.[13] We should expect that the greater the latitude in allowing the dentists in a state to delegate tasks the greater the hourly earnings of dentists in that state will be.

The principal auxiliaries affected by the "expanded-duty" developments are the dental hygienist and the dental assistant. The expansion of their allowed duties has occurred either through an "open provision for" or a "list of" new expanded duties.

An "open provision" for expanded duties presents a flexible definition of the expanded-duty auxiliary's new role. Under this provision, the dentist is allowed to assign the auxiliary any task for which he believes the auxiliary is suitably trained, subject either to a list of duties which the auxiliary is prohibited from performing, or a general restriction against the auxiliary's performing duties which require the knowledge and skill of a dentist.

A "list" of functions allowed the expanded-duty auxiliary, on the other hand, provides a much less flexible definition of the new role. The functions on the list, and only those functions, may be performed. The dentist is not at liberty to allow the auxiliary to perform tasks other than those on the list even if he believes the auxiliary is capable of performing them.

Of course, many states have no provision for expanded-duty auxiliaries, and even those that do may provide differently for the expansion of hygienists' duties from the way they provide for the expansion of assistants' duties. Some states, for example, allow for an expanded-duty hygienist but not an expanded-duty assistant.

Some may have an "open provision" for assistants' duties and a "list" for the hygienists' duties.

It may be expected that a dentist's practice will be more productive the easier it is for him to delegate tasks which can be performed by less highly trained personnel; that is, his hourly earnings will be higher if he spends his hours doing the work of a dentist rather than the work of a dentist's assistant. We may construct a dummy variable measure of the extent to which the dentist is allowed such delegation: if the state has no provision for expanded-duty personnel, the state is assigned a value of zero; if the state has a list of expanded duties, the state is assigned a value of unity; if the state has an open provision for expanded-duty personnel, the state is assigned a value of two. Thus, the dummy variable for each type of auxiliary takes on the values zero, one and two. The sum of the dummy variables for auxiliaries and for hygienists is defined to be a measure of the extent to which the dentist is free to delegate tasks. The sum can take on the values zero, one, two, three and four. The hourly earnings of dentists are expected to be positively related to this dummy variable.

Other Factors To Be Held Constant. In order to isolate the effect of these two specific regulatory factors on the earnings of dentists, it is necessary to hold constant (control for) the effects of other important factors that influence a dentist's hourly earnings. These variables are described briefly below.

Experience. For the dentist (as for many other workers), the greater the amount of his labor force experience, the higher his hourly earnings are likely to be, inasmuch as a considerable amount of training takes place on the job in dentistry as in other occupations.[14] After a certain point in life, however, all the effects of on-the-job learning have generally been absorbed so that the effect of the general deterioration of skills and abilities with age begins to predominate: hourly earnings may begin to decline as a result of this reduced productivity. Consequently, both experience and its square are entered as separate variables in the analysis to provide for this possible parabolic pattern of hourly earnings according to experience. It should be noted here that the absence of recently graduated dentists (excluded from the sample) may make it difficult for us to observe the relation between experience and earnings.

Education. Dentists with more years of education than the average are expected to have higher than average hourly earnings.[15] Since dentists with more than average education may be either specialists or general practitioners who attended college for a longer time before entering dental school, it is important to point out that even the additional years of undergraduate college may be expected to generate higher hourly earnings for the dentist.

Per Capita Incomes. The demand for dental services is greater the greater the incomes of the individual consumers of dental care. Unless the dental market is always in equilibrium, the earnings of dentists can be expected to be higher the higher the per capita incomes where the dentists are located. Per capita incomes in a state may also be considered as an indicator of living costs in the state; in this case also, they would be expected to be positively related to the earnings of dentists.

Dentists Per 100,000 Population. Dentists in states with relatively few dentists per 100,000 people, other factors being held constant, may be expected to have higher earnings, since they may charge higher prices for the same quantity of services provided in states with more dentists per 100,000 people.

Self-Employment Status. Whether a dentist is self-employed (self-employed dentists constitute 96 percent of all dentists in the sample) may be expected to affect his hourly earnings. Self-employed dentists, who receive returns to their entrepreneurial talent and to the capital investment in their offices, should be expected to have higher hourly earnings than employee dentists. (It should be noted that there may be a small bias in the self-employment-status variable.)[16]

The Empirical Results. The results of this investigation appear in Appendix D. The results indicate that experience is significantly parabolically related to earnings and that education is significantly positively related to earnings, as was anticipated. Self-employed dentists have hourly earnings that are significantly higher than employee dentists (by $3.35 per hour). The number of dentists per 100,000 people in the civilian population in the state is negatively related to hourly earnings, but the relationship is not significant. Per capita income is positively related to hourly earnings, but the relationship is also not significant.

Allowing the dentist to delegate more tasks produces a significant increase in his hourly earnings. Dentists in states with an "open provision" for both assistants and hygienists earned $1.68 more per hour (or $3,746 annually, given an average of 2,230 hours worked per year) than dentists in states with no provision for expanded-duty auxiliaries. Dentists in states with a "list" of expanded duties for both these auxiliaries earned $.84 more per hour (or $1,873 more per year) than dentists in states with no provisions for expanded-duty personnel.

The average failure rate on the licensure examination for the previous decade is significantly and positively related to hourly earnings. In a state with an average failure rate (for the 1960–1969 decade) amounting to ten percentage points (one standard deviation) above the U.S. average of 14 percent, dentists earned $.70 more per hour ($1,561 more per year) than in states with the average failure rate.

Summary

The evidence, though not conclusive, suggests that dentists can and do benefit from the licensing powers granted to them by the states. By restricting entry into the profession, dentists increase their hourly earnings. By allowing expanded-duty auxiliaries, the dentists also increase their hourly earnings. In the latter case, consumers can also benefit from lower prices which competition among the more productive dentists produces.

In view of the advantages to dentists that would accrue from allowing the use of expanded-duty auxiliaries, it is difficult to understand why movement in that direction has not been more rapid. One study suggests that resistance to this change can be explained by the composition of the members of the state licensing boards.

State laws ensure that many dental licensing boards will be composed entirely of older and more experienced dentists. Board members generally must have been in practice for at least five or ten years and, in some cases, that figure must represent continuous practice in the state. In addition, board members are generally selected from a list of nominees submitted by the state dental association. The nominees are likely to be older well-known practitioners in the state. (Younger practitioners are apparently more receptive to the idea of using expanded-duty auxiliaries than are older practitioners.) Moreover, board members generally are not allowed to be affiliated with a dental school; familiarity with new techniques would, of course, likely be greater among those dentists affiliated with a dental school than among those not so affiliated. The use of expanded-duty auxiliaries may be seen as a threat to the dentist's traditional role by those dentists who are unfamiliar with and unreceptive to the new technique. Unless they conform to the new techniques, the older well-established dentists are likely to lose business to practices with expanded-duty personnel that can treat more patients per hour and at a lower price than practices without expanded-duty personnel.[17] In view of the fact that expanded-duty personnel can provide additional services without any reduction in the quality of services provided,[18] the loss of business could be substantial once consumers learn of the advantages of service where these expanded-duty personnel were used.

The prospect of altering the licensing system which produces such results as these is not very promising. Judicial intervention on the basis of due process violation or the violation of antitrust laws is not likely to take place on behalf of those auxiliaries who wish to perform expanded duties. Extensive alterations are more likely to occur through changes in the statutes. Alteration of state laws to change the composition of the licensing boards and the definition and function of auxiliary personnel is likely to be the major road to change in the licensing system.[19] In this connection, it might be appropriate for the federal government to consider becoming involved in establishing uniform and reasonable regulatory policies at the state level.[20]

CHAPTER V

THE RATIONALE FOR GOVERNMENT INTERVENTION

The legislative history of the student loan and scholarship program and the formula grant program suggests that the legislators did not have a clear and consistent policy in mind when the legislation was drafted. The fact that the interest rate charged on student loans was first set at the long-term federal debt rate, then fixed at 3 percent, and more recently fixed at 7 percent, would suggest uncertainty as to whether students were to receive a subsidy by paying a rate below the market level for long-term loans. The fact that the scholarship program, first established for students from low-income families, and then redefined to be for students in exceptional financial need, has been considered for termination also indicates uncertainty as to whether dental students should receive a subsidy. The fact that the formula grant program to dental schools, conceived to prevent an imminent financial collapse of the nation's dental schools, may now become essentially a student loan program likewise indicates the uncertainty that has prevailed as to whether it is appropriate to subsidize dental schools.

It is important, therefore, for us to consider the various alternative explanations for government involvement in the dental care market so as to determine what kind of action is justified.

Externalities or Neighborhood Effects

Whenever the production or consumption of a commodity by one individual or agent in the economy creates a cost or bestows a benefit directly upon someone else without compensation, an externality is said to exist.[1] Air pollution is an example of an external cost produced by the operation of an automobile or an oil refinery, or an electrical power plant. Water pollution is another example of an external cost produced by the operation of various industries—paper manufacture, for example—and waste treatment facilities.

Because property rights in air and water are defined as communal property rights, the air and water belong to everyone—which may be another way of saying they belong to no one. In cases such as these, it is necessary for the government to enforce the communal property rights and collect revenues in order to clean up the air or water. Whenever the administrative cost proves to be low enough, the government attempts to require those who are responsible for producing the externality to pay for the cleanup in proportion to their contribution to the problem. Hence, government may impose taxes on autos for their emissions and on plants for their discharge of wastes. These taxes take the form of requiring the installation of devices to reduce or eliminate the discharge of wastes.

In the case of medicine, the most obvious form of externality is the cost of epidemic disease. If one person's having an untreated case of smallpox means that others with whom he comes in contact will also develop smallpox, then that person is the source of an important external cost. Others have a right to insist they not be exposed to the risk of smallpox. One solution is to isolate the diseased person—thus, houses in the past were "quarantined" if a member of the household had an epidemic disease. Once a vaccine for smallpox became available, however, the external cost of the epidemic disease could be eliminated by prevention. The United States government eventually required that everyone be vaccinated against smallpox. Costs of enforcement were not prohibitively large since entry into school and entry of persons from abroad could be made conditional upon vaccination. The smallpox vaccination program was financed out of general revenues at the state and federal level. This country's recent experience with polio is another example of the treatment of an external cost in medicine.[2]

It is difficult to discover any external costs in the dental care market. There are no known epidemic dental diseases. The cost of community water fluoridation is more properly viewed as a transfer payment than as an externality, since the existence of fluoridation tablets (which can be purchased by a family and placed in water used for drinking in the home) suggests that the issue is not the existence of an external cost or benefit but rather the desire to obtain fluoridated water at a lower cost than fluoridation tablets would produce. The opponents of community fluoridation correctly point out that an external cost is being generated for them by the fluoridation of the community's water supply. Until recently, there was no way to eliminate this external cost concomitant with community fluoridation. With the development of filters which eliminate virtually all of the fluoride placed in the water and which can be inserted into the faucets of the homes not wishing to drink fluoridated water, the issue is more clearly drawn. Those favoring fluoridation can afford to pay for the installation of such filters in the home of every fluoridation opponent and still be far better off than they would be if they had to purchase the fluoride tablets.[3]

Aside from dental care externalities that give rise to questions of income redistribution—these are dealt with in the last section of this chapter—it would seem that the most important dental care externality arises in connection with dental research. Dental research is similar to other forms of research in that once the knowledge has been generated, it is extremely difficult, if not impossible, for the person who made the discovery to prevent others from benefitting from it. Once a profitable idea has been discovered, it can easily be transmitted and used by others. The development of copyright and patent laws in this country are an attempt to provide a kind of "property right" in new ideas and techniques; those who hold copyrights or patents are able to benefit from the sale of their "property" and have an incentive to develop new ideas and techniques. However, the great difficulty in establishing "priority" and "originality" has made the patent and copyright laws subject to litigation which has undoubtedly reduced the incentive to conduct research.[4]

Because research activity may involve an important externality that is frequently difficult to internalize by patent grants, governments have more and more been viewed as the appropriate vehicles for promoting research activity. The benefits of dental research activity, for example, are bestowed upon society in general; it is argued that society should therefore be willing to pay to insure that dental research is conducted. That is, indeed, what this society (through its federal dental research establishment) has done.

Imperfect Capital Markets

The capital market—that is, the market for loanable funds—is sometimes said to be operating imperfectly.[5] Moreover, it is said to operate less perfectly with regard to human than physical capital.[6]

The successful operation of the private market is defined by competition to provide goods and services at the lowest possible cost. Competition requires that it be easy for firms to enter an attractive industry—which means, among other things, that firms must be able to borrow sufficient amounts of money to acquire the needed machinery to begin production. If the financial intermediaries who should do the lending are not able to do it, then entry becomes more difficult and competition is reduced.

It is widely recognized that borrowing for the purpose of acquiring human capital is sometimes difficult. One important reason for this is that the lending agency seldom is offered any collateral for such a loan: the borrower, usually a young adult with few assets of his own, has nothing to offer except the likelihood of his repaying the loan. In our society he cannot offer his own future services as collateral—he cannot sell himself. In the event of default, the lender would have little recourse for recovering his loan except to sue for whatever assets the student acquired during and after training.[7] In this situation a lender is likely to lend only to those students who are virtually certain to acquire their human capital, to have the earnings in the future to repay the loan and the incentive to do so. In other words, loans are likely to be made only to those students who represent the very best credit risks. A student's parents can underwrite the loan, of course, and this improves the student's chances of obtaining a loan. It does not, however, ensure equal access to the capital markets, since not all students have parents who are in a position to underwrite their loan.

In recognition of this difficulty in the human capital market, this country has developed a number of student loan programs designed to insure the private lender against default. The National Defense Education Act provided a loan program, of this sort, combined with a subsidy to lower the interest rate paid by the student. This program is available to students attending graduate and professional schools.

It is not clear that a federal loan program for dental students is really needed, inasmuch as dental students are considered good credit risks and can obtain loans in the private financial markets. Data presented in Table 9 indicate that in the 1972–1973 academic year dental students in the United States were able to obtain nearly $3 million in loans from banks, out of the total of nearly $15 million they borrowed. In addition, they obtained over $800,000 from universities, over $900,000 from a dental association, and over $600,000 from additional sources other than the federal or state governments. That is to say, it appears that more than one-third of dental student loans came from sources other than federal or state government. The situation was similar in the 1971–1972 academic year.

Table 9

AMOUNT AND SOURCE OF LOAN FUNDS FOR DENTAL STUDENTS, BY SOURCE

		Source					
Academic Year	**Total**	Federal	State	University	Bank	Dental association	Other
1973–74	$20,954,587	$10,417,678	$2,839,334	$4,880,142			$2,817,433
1972–73	14,913,344	8,009,367	1,650,069	807,349	$2,914,680	$908,409	623,470
1971–72	12,230,529	7,480,590	1,121,637	563,362	2,167,645	417,589	479,706
1969–70	6,881,582 [a]	4,707,083		2,174,499			
1968–69	7,215,543 [a]	8,054,449		1,161,094			

[a] These figures represent the total loans available from federal and university sources and are not necessarily the total of all loan funds available.

Source: Council on Dental Education, American Dental Association, *Annual Report*, various years (1968-69 data from 1969/70 report, p. 19; 1969-70 data from 1970/71 report, p. 33; and data for 1971/72, 1972/73, and 1973/74 from reports for those years, p. 35, p. 17, and p. 17, respectively). Data for 1970-71 were not collected.

Imperfect Information

Another major reason for government intervention in the marketplace is that consumers may lack adequate, reliable information concerning the price and quality of the products they are buying or want to buy.[8] A competitive dental market is assumed to consist of well-informed and reasonable mobile consumers who possess adequate information on the price, quantity, and quality of all the dental goods and services available for sale in the market. The argument that the consumer is not and perhaps cannot be well informed about the purchase of medical care has been one basis for the licensing of health practitioners generally, dentists among them.[9] Licensing, by providing that only "high" quality services are offered for sale, is supposed to provide the consumer with the information he needs. High quality care, of course, is expensive, but it is argued that this added expense is less than the cost of bad quality service for the consumer. The argument is particularly applicable to medical procedures that are either irreversible or fatal in the event of error. The danger of licensing is, of course, that the licensing authority will be used to provide more expensive but not necessarily higher quality care to the medical consumer.

Since dentistry, unlike medicine, involves relatively few irreversible or fatal procedures, the case for licensing is not so strong. There would, however, likely be a high cost to repeated trial and error in finding good quality dental care; it appears that this high cost is one possible explanation for providing the consumer with information through licensing. It might, however, be possible to eliminate this cost in another way, involving certification of dentists by the existing licensing boards, which would test and grade applicants: the boards would "certify" those who passed, but not prevent those who failed from practicing, though it would prevent their use of the term "certified" along with their name. This should accomplish the same objective. Moreover, restraints on advertising could be removed. Advertising does serve to provide information to consumers, in addition to trying to persuade them. In short, there are other ways of resolving information problems besides licensing.

Income Redistribution

Perhaps the government's principal concern for externalities in the dental care market is a concern with redistribution of income in the form of resources to purchase dental care. For despite the term "insurance," the national dental insurance programs now being considered really represent various ways of accomplishing an income transfer of a certain kind to certain groups of people in the economy. Because of the high probability of small losses and the existence of "moral hazard," dental care is simply not a likely market for insurance.[10]

The target groups for Medicare and Medicaid programs are the elderly and the poor, respectively. Our society has decided it would like to eliminate the sight of old or poor people suffering from illnesses which they are unable to treat because of their low incomes and the high price of treatment. Moreover, we have decided we are willing to expend resources to accomplish that objective. The healthier individuals in our society can be thought of as experiencing an external cost when they see or hear about old or poor people who are sick and unable to buy medical services. This cost occurs because the welfare of a given individual depends not only upon the quantity of goods and services he himself consumes but also upon the quantities of certain goods and services (such as medical services) consumed by certain others (such as old and poor people).[11]

There are several ways to accomplish the transfer of health resources to old and poor people. One is simply to increase their incomes sufficiently to enable them to buy the health resources they would otherwise be unable to buy. This would allow old and poor people to purchase goods and services other than medical goods and services if they so desired. Since it is their ill health that gives rise to the desire to help them, not their inability to purchase other goods and services (for which society has a Social Security program to transfer financial resources to old people and welfare programs to transfer other goods and services to poor people), general income transfers are not considered the best way to accomplish the objective. Another way of accomplishing this transfer—and this would accomplish only the desired transfer—would be to provide free medical care to old and poor people. But this has the disadvantage that old and poor people would have no incentive to economize on the use of this medical care. As long as the medical care provides them some positive benefit, it is argued, they tend to make use of it, thus straining the available medical resources which must serve other sick people as well.[12] The cost of this approach to the problem could thus be quite high.

Still another way of accomplishing the transfer involves subsidizing the price which old or poor people pay for their health services. This is similar to the approach being used today to transfer resources for food to poor people through the food stamp program.

This approach would enable old and poor people to purchase more health services than they would otherwise purchase and yet give them an incentive to use those resources wisely by requiring them to pay a portion of the bills. The analysis presented in Chapter 3 indicates that even this approach would be costly; a universal 20 percent copayment program would more or less double total expenditures on dental care in the United States. Some would argue, moreover, that this approach makes it difficult to accomplish the program's objectives, since the low incomes of old and poor people make them unable to afford medical care at even these subsidized prices.[13] An additional problem resides in the location of offices administering the income transfer program and the location of the program's intended beneficiaries; the nearer the office to the intended beneficiaries, the greater the participation in the program.[14]

Summary

In brief, it may be said that the presence of externalities in dental research explains government involvement in dental research, the presence of externalities in income distribution explains transfer programs such as Medicaid (which applies to dentistry), and the existence of imperfect information provides a reason for the certification of dentists and should insure that advertising be allowed in the dental care market. Such programs as the dental student scholarship program, the formula grant program to dental schools, the construction grant-in-aid program to dental schools, and the subsidy of the interest rate on dental student loans cannot be explained on these grounds. These programs do not appear to be appropriate forms for government action to take.[15] Even the government loan programs to dental students are questionable inasmuch as dental students are good credit risks and have access to private lending institutions.

The licensing of dentists and other dental personnel would appear to be inappropriately strong action for government at the state level: certification, with advertising, would satisfy the need for providing consumers with the information they need about the quality of care they can obtain in the dental care market.

To some extent, some of the recently proposed changes in the federal programs are encouraging. The phasing out of the unconditional scholarship program, the replacement of the formula program grant by what is in effect a loan program, and the increasing of the interest rate on student loans to a level nearer current market rates would all be important steps in the direction of improving the efficiency of the dental care market. Considerable expense to the taxpayers could have been avoided by more careful consideration of the issues involved—and of these actions—at the time the programs were initiated.

CHAPTER VI

SUMMARY AND CONCLUSIONS

The involvement of the federal government in the programs designed to increase the supply of dentists through various forms of subsidy has been unnecessary and inappropriate—and, moreover, costly. The government has provided loans and scholarships to students who did not need loans and scholarships and who in any case could generally have obtained them without government action. Only a small fraction of the students receiving scholarships would have failed to enroll in a dental school in the absence of scholarship aid. In view of the financial attractiveness of becoming a dentist (the rate of return on dentists' training amounted to over 25 percent in 1970, and the average net earnings for a dentist in 1973 amounted to $34,455), it is difficult to see why additional incentive would need to be provided by the federal government. And in view of the fact that the typical dental student is considered a good credit risk by private lending institutions, it is not at all clear why the federal government should be involved in a dental student loan program.

The government has assisted in the construction of facilities designed to create additional places for dental school students; many of these places would have been created anyway. This construction program, like the scholarship program, has been extraordinarily expensive and provided only modest results. Not only has the cost of each dental school place created by the program been about twice what it has previously been calculated to be, but even according to previous calculations, the cost per place created was a sizable $154,942.

Despite the evident wastefulness of these government programs, and despite the high costs of a care program such as Medicaid, there is pressure for the creation of an expensive universal dental care program on a national level. If we assume a copayment level of 20 percent, we find—using our simple economic model—that in 1970 federal expenditures on such a program (in 1970 dollars) would have been almost $10 billion, roughly speaking, and might under certain circumstances have been more than $10 billion. Of course, federal expenditures would vary according to the copayment percentage, according to what age and income groups are covered, and according to what kinds of treatment are covered by such a program.

Since the evidence, though it is not conclusive, does suggest that dentists may benefit from the licensing powers granted them by the states, we might profitably consider a change in these powers or in the composition of licensing boards as an alternative to new federal programs. By restricting entry into the profession, dentists increase their hourly earnings. But by allowing expanded-duty auxiliaries, they may also increase their hourly earnings, while at the same time reducing the cost of dental care, since consumers can benefit from the lower prices which competition among the more productive dentists will create.

Greater use of expanded-duty auxiliaries, along with efforts to increase the availability of fluoridated water (to those who want it), could reduce federal expenditures by at least $500 million and perhaps $1.1 billion annually (1970 figures), bringing down prices while increasing the amount of dental services available. In view of the advantages that would accrue both to the dentists and to the public from the use of expanded-duty auxiliaries, it must be concluded that the failure of the dental profession to move rapidly toward the fuller use of these auxiliaries is traceable to the composition of the dental licensing boards. State laws generally guarantee that these boards will be composed of older and more experienced dentists, not affiliated with dental schools, and therefore on two counts (age and what might be called "insularity") unlikely to welcome the innovation represented by the expanded-duty auxiliary.

The likelihood of an alteration in the licensing system is not great. Judicial intervention might, of course, take place on the basis of due-process or antitrust violations, but this does not appear very likely. Statutory changes are more likely than judicial intervention—in fact, changes in state laws to change the composition of the licensing boards and the definition and function of auxiliary personnel represent the probable road to overall change. It might be appropriate for the federal government to intervene to establish uniform and reasonable regulatory policies at the state level.

It is difficult to accept many of the other reasons given for government intervention in dental care. Granted, the presence of externalities in dental research explains government involvement in dental research, though the externalities are not great. The presence of externalities in income distribution explains transfer programs such as Medicaid (which applies to dental care), though it does not of course justify the high costs of Medicaid. The existence of imperfect information provides a reason for the certification of dentists (as for the certification of accountants), though not necessarily for their licensing, and it would seem that imperfect information would also provide a reason for dentists to advertise—though state laws or regulations generally do not permit professional advertisement. But such programs as the dental student scholarship program, the formula grant program to dental schools, the construction grant-in-aid program for dental schools, and the interest-rate subsidy to dental students cannot be justified on these grounds, or indeed on any grounds. Moreover, the licensing of dentists and other dental personnel would appear to be inappropriately strong action on the part of the states: certification with advertising would satisfy the need for providing consumers with the requisite information on the quality of dental care they can obtain.

The appropriate form of government action on the supply side would be an end to the control that dentists have, by virtue of state licensing laws, over the number and size of dental schools and the nature and organization of dental practice. By replacing existing licensing laws with certification procedures which would "grade" dentists, dental auxiliaries, and dental schools, but would not prevent "ungraded" or "low-grade" dentists, dental auxiliaries, and dental schools from continuing activity, the government would provide consumers with more dental services than they have now at a lower price than they have now, at the same time it provided the necessary information for them to make choices on quality of service.

APPENDIX

APPENDIX A: SPECIFICATIONS OF THE VARIOUS HPEA LOAN, SCHOLARSHIP, CONSTRUCTION AND FORMULA GRANT EXPENDITURES

The Health Professions Educational Assistance Act (HPEA, Public Law 88–129) initially established a three-year program of loans of up to $2,000 per year to be made at interest rates comparable to the yield on long-term federal debt obligations (but not to be less than 3 percent per year) and having a ten year term beginning three years after graduation.[1] The Health Professions Educational Assistance Amendments of 1965 (Public Law 89–290) extended the loan program for another three years and increased the maximum loan amount to $2,500 per year. These amendments provided that any student of medicine, dentistry, or optometry who practiced in a shortage area would be forgiven 10 percent of his loan for every year of such practice up to a maximum of five years. These amendments also established a scholarship program of up to $2,500 per student per year for students from low-income families. The total of scholarship grants to any school was limited to $2,000 times 10 percent of the number of full-time students.[2]

The Health Manpower Act of 1968 (Public Law 90–490) extended the loan and scholarship program for another two years, fixed the interest rate for the loan program at 3 percent per year and required repayment to begin one year after graduation, unless advanced training (including internships and residencies) were undertaken in which case repayment would begin upon completion of such training. The 1968 act redefined student eligibility for scholarship aid to be "exceptional financial need," instead of being from a low-income family.[3] The Comprehensive Health Manpower Training Act of 1971 (Public Law 92–157) extended the loan program for another three years, increased the maximum loan or scholarship amount from $2,500 to $3,500 per student per year and added a forgiveness provision for loans to students from low-income or disadvantaged families who did not complete their studies. The act also amended the shortage-area loan forgiveness program to provide for 30 percent per year forgiveness for the first two years and 25 percent for the third year of practice in a shortage area, for practice of at least two years in such an area. The total of scholarship grants to any school was limited to $3,000 (up from $2,000) times either the number of full-time students or the number of such students from low-income backgrounds, whichever was greater.[4]

In 1974, both the Senate and the House considered differing legislation which would have altered the loan program by increasing the interest rate from 3 to 7 percent and by redefining the maximum loan amount per student per year to be $2,500 plus tuition costs instead of $3,500. The legislation would have provided for phasing out the unconditional scholarship program and would have replaced it with increased funding of the National Health Service Corps scholarship program, modified to provide a release from all service obligations to students who agreed to practice in a critical health shortage area upon graduation for as many years as they received scholarship aid. The amount of each year's Service Corps scholarship would consist of basic pay and allowances of a commissioned officer on active duty in the Service Corps plus tuition and expenses.[5] Since no law emerged from the Congress in 1974, existing programs are being funded at previous levels while Congress reconsiders health manpower legislation in 1975.

Responsibility for the distribution of loan and scholarship funds was left to the participating schools. Participating schools were required to contribute 10 percent of the money for the loan program initially, but later they were offered the option of issuing promissory notes for repayment to the federal government. For any one year schools were allowed to transfer to a loan fund up to 20 percent of the money received for the scholarship program if the school provided 10 percent of the money to the loan fund. Transfers to the scholarship program from such a loan fund were also allowed.[6] Transfers to and from a loan fund for which the school provided no portion were not allowed.[7] The determination of student eligibility for either loan or scholarship assistance was left to the participating school; but to qualify for scholarship assistance a student was supposed to have exceptional financial need. In determining need, participating schools were to consider the cost of attending school in relation to the financial resources available to the student and his parents.[8]

Federal grants for school construction costs were initially limited to 50 percent of the costs, although payments amounting to two-thirds of construction costs were allowed in cases where a major expansion was involved. The 1968 act allowed the federal share to rise to two-thirds when this rise was necessary for the school to complete the construction program. The 1971 act increased the federal share to 70 percent or up to 80 percent for new schools, major expansions or schools located in shortage areas.[9] The legislation considered in 1974 would have increased the federal share to 80 percent in general.[10]

Under the 1965 act formula grants were initially limited to $12,500 per school plus $250 times the number of full-time students, increasing to $25,000 per school plus $500 times the number of full-time students by 1967. The 1971 act increased the formula to $2,500 for each first, second and third year student, plus $1,000 for each bonus enrollment student, plus $1,000 for each student training as a physician assistant or dental therapist, plus $4,000 for each student completing studies in more than three years, plus $6,000 for each student completing studies in three years or less.[11] The legislation considered in 1974 defined the formula to be $2,100 per student per year, declining to $2,000 per student per year in three years; 25 percent of this money was to be spent for training students during their third and fourth years at remote sites for at least six weeks in each year. In addition, the school would receive $650 for each full-time student enrolled in a physician-assistant or expanded-duty dental auxiliary program, provided the school agreed to expand enrollment by a specified amount. But, for the first time, each school receiving support through a formula would have been required to sign a contract with each enrolled student whereby the student agreed to pay back to the federal government in annual installments the amount the school received in support for each student.[12] Thus, support through the formula would have become a loan program to the student.

Funds would also have been made available under this legislation for identifying and enrolling disadvantaged students, establishing area health education centers, training personnel in emergency medical services, computer technology, health care demonstration programs, remedial training of U.S. citizen graduates of foreign medical schools, establishing departments of family medicine, and other special projects.[13]

APPENDIX B: RATES OF RETURN AND DENTAL ENROLLMENTS

Two basic equations were estimated from the data in Table 4:

$$\frac{\overline{E}_{t+1}}{\overline{B}_{t+1}} = a + b\,\frac{R_t}{i_t} \tag{1}$$

$$\frac{A_{t+1}}{B_{t+1}} = c + d\,\frac{R_t}{i_t} \tag{2}$$

where $\overline{E}$ is the average size of the freshman dental school class during the period of years from $t+1$ to $t+3$ following an observation on the rate of return in year t, $\overline{B}$ is the average annual number of earned bachelor's and first degrees in the physical and biological sciences during the same period, A_{t+1} is the number of applicants to dental school in year $t+1$, B_{t+1} is the number of earned bachelor's and first degrees in the physical and biological sciences in year $t+1$, R_t is the rate of return on investment in dental training in year t, and i_t is the yield in year t on U.S. government securities of ten-to-fifteen years duration. The regression results are presented in Table B–1 in equations (1) and (2) in linear form and in equations (3) and (4) in log form. As is evident from a comparison of the equations, the one for applicants in each case explains more of the variance and has a higher elasticity with respect to the independent variable R_t/i_t than the one for students enrolled. The Durbin-Watson statistic indicates that autocorrelation is not a problem, although this is an inference from an extrapolation of existing Durbin-Watson tables for sample sizes below fifteen. Autocorrelation, though it produces unbiased regression coefficients, can result in serious understatement of the sampling variances for the regression coefficients and for the residuals. Significant results could thus be obtained when there is no significant relation present. As a precaution, therefore, Table B–1 presents the Cochrane-Orcutt estimates, which corrects for this variance understatement, for each of the four equations. The estimate of the first-order autocorrelation coefficient is insignificant in all cases, indicating that first-order correlation is

Table B-1
TESTING FOR POSSIBLE AUTOCORRELATION

Equation	R^2	F	Durbin-Watson	Elasticity	N	P
(1) $\frac{\bar{E}}{\bar{B}} = .035 + \underset{(2.44)^{*}}{.015} \frac{R_t}{i_t}$	.50	5.96*	1.53	.69	8	
(2) $\frac{A_{t+1}}{B_{t+1}} = .058 + \underset{(4.09)^{**}}{.035} \frac{R_t}{i_t}$	.74	16.71**	2.61	.76	8	
(3) $Ln \frac{(\bar{E})}{(\bar{B})} = 3.27 + \underset{(2.25)^{*}}{.654} \, Ln \frac{(R_t)}{(i_t)}$	.46	5.04*	1.32	.65	8	
(4) $Ln \frac{(A_{t+1})}{(B_{t+1})} = -2.67 + \underset{(4.13)^{**}}{.752} \, Ln \frac{(R_t)}{(i_t)}$	.74	17.07**	2.32	.75	8	
Cochrane-Orcutt Estimates						
(1)′ $\frac{\bar{E}}{\bar{B}} = .007 + \underset{(2.95)^{**}}{.021} \frac{R_t}{i_t}$	.65	9.21**	1.35	.98	7	.039 (.08)
(2)′ $\frac{A_{t+1}}{B_{t+1}} = .076 + \underset{(3.99)^{**}}{.031} \frac{R_t}{i_t}$	.63	8.42*	1.37	.72	7	−.320 (−.91)
(3)′ $Ln \frac{(\bar{E})}{(\bar{B})} = -3.30 + \underset{(1.62)\#}{.695} \, Ln \frac{(R_t)}{(i_t)}$	.54	5.90*	1.18	.70	7	.267 (.73)
(4)′ $Ln \frac{(A_{t+1})}{(B_{t+1})} = -2.55 + \underset{(3.40)^{*}}{.665} \, Ln \frac{(R_t)}{(i_t)}$	.62	8.25*	1.55	.67	7	−.17 (−.46)

Notes: *t*-statistics are in parentheses; * means significant at the 5 percent level (two-tailed *t*-test); ** means significant at the 1 percent level (two-tailed *t*-test); # means significant at the 10 percent level (one-tailed *t*-test).

Table B-1 (Continued)

Definitions of Variables: $\bar{E}$—average size of freshman dental school class during period $t+1$ to $t+3$; R_t—rate of return to dentists in year t assuming (.6, .1) draft probabilities for dentists and college graduates, respectively, for all years except 1952 and 1967 when (.9, .2) is assumed; $\bar{B}$—average annual earned bachelor's and first degrees in the physical and biological sciences in the U.S. during period $t+1$ to $t+3$; B_{t+1}—earned bachelor's and first degrees in the physical and biological sciences in year $t+1$; A_{t+1}—applicants to dental school in year $t+1$; i_t—yield on U.S. government securities of ten to fifteen year duration in year t.

Sources: *E*—Council on Dental Education, *Dental Student Register* and *Annual Report on Dental Education* (American Dental Association, 211 East Chicago Avenue, Chicago, Illinois, 1950–1974). *R*—Alex Maurizi, *Economic Essays on the Dental Profession* (University of Iowa, Iowa City, 1969), p. 13; the three most recent rates have been calculated by the author but not published. *B*—"Earned Degrees Conferred by Field of Study and Level of Degree," *U.S. Statistical Abstract*, 1948–1974. *i*—*Economic Report of the President 1973*, p. 260.

not present. Moreover, the significance of the results is only slightly altered by the Cochrane-Orcutt adjustment. For further details on the Cochrane-Orcutt procedure, see J. Johnston, *Econometric Methods* (New York: McGraw-Hill, 1972), p. 262.

APPENDIX C: THE TWO-STAGE ESTIMATION PROCEDURE USED IN THE TWO-EQUATION MODEL IN CHAPTER 3

Our relatively simple two-equation linear model is displayed in equations (1) and (2) below. Enclosed in parentheses are signs indicating the expected relation between the variables on the right-hand side of the equation and the variable on the left-hand side.

$$\text{Demand:}\quad Q = a + \overset{(-)}{bP} + \overset{(+)}{cPCY} + \overset{(-)}{dFL} \tag{1}$$

$$\text{Supply:}\quad Q = e + \underset{(+)}{fP} + \underset{(+)}{gK} = \underset{(+)}{hAX} + \underset{(+)}{jHRS} \tag{2}$$

The variables for this model were measured in the following way. *Q*, the quantity of dental services, is measured by the annual number of patient sittings for the dental practice. *P*, the price of dental services, is measured by the price of a patient sitting, approximated by the dentist's gross annual income divided by his annual patient sittings. *PCY*, the level of consumer income, is measured by the average per capita personal income of all individuals in the state in which the dentist's practice is located. *FL*, the extent of fluoridation, is measured by the percent of the population in the state drinking fluoridated water (either natural fluoridated or controlled fluoridated water). *K* is the number of chairs in the office. *AX* is the number of full-time auxiliaries. *HRS* is the annual number of hours worked by the dentist.

The two-equation model has two endogenous variables, *P* and *Q*, and five exogenous variables, *PCY*, *FL*, *K*, *AX* and *HRS*. It is exactly identified: that is, there are as many unknown variables (two) to be solved for in the model as there are equations. The reason for using a two-stage estimation procedure is to eliminate the correlation between the disturbance term and the endogenous variable on the right-hand side (in this case, *P*) which disrupts the estimates obtained by direct application of ordinary least squares to the model equations. The first stage eliminates this correlation by estimating *P* with the five exogenous variables; the second stage replaces *P* with the estimated value of P in each equation of the model and then estimates these with ordinary least squares. For further details, the reader is referred to Johnston, *Econometric Methods*, pp. 380–384. The method is illustrated below.

Stage I: $P = a + bPCY + cFL + dK + eAX + fHRS$

This equation is estimated with ordinary least squares. The resulting estimate, P', is used in Stage II.

Stage II: $Q = u + vP' + wPCY + xFL$
$Q = m + nP' + rK + sAX + tHRS$

Each of these equations is estimated with ordinary least squares. The results are presented in equations (3) and (4) below. Displayed below each regression coefficient is its standard error.[1] The results are as expected; each coefficient has the expected sign and is significantly greater than its standard error.

$$\frac{\text{Demand:}}{F = 26} \quad Q = 6596 - \underset{(61)}{446P} + \underset{(.19)}{1.64PCY} - \underset{(5)}{36FL} \tag{3}$$

$$\frac{\text{Supply:}}{F = 150} \quad Q = -514 + \underset{(14)}{51P} + \underset{(42)}{377K} + \underset{(47)}{509AX} + \underset{(.06)}{.83HRS} \tag{4}$$

$N = 2309$

P = price of dental services
Q = quantity of dental services
PCY = consumer income
FL = extent of fluoridation
K = number of chairs in the office
AX = number of full-time auxiliaries
HRS = number of hours worked annually by the dentist

Equilibrium in the absence of an insurance program is determined by solving equations (3) and (4) for P and Q (endogenous variables) in terms of all of the other (exogenous) variables, namely PCY, FL, K, AX, and HRS. Equating (3) and (4), since the quantity of sittings demanded must equal the quantity of sittings supplied in equilibrium, and solving this, we come to the reduced-form equations (5) and (6) below.

$$\overline{P} = 14.3 + .003PCY - .07FL - .76K - 1.02AX - .002HRS \tag{5}$$

$$\overline{Q} = 2.8 + .30PCY - 4.8FL + 339K + 455AX + .89HRS \tag{6}$$

Briefly, these reduced-form equations indicate that equilibrium prices and quantities, shown as $\overline{P}$ and $\overline{Q}$, are a function of the variables which shift the positions of the demand and supply equations. A rise in incomes would shift the demand curve outward, to the right, for example, and result in higher prices and greater quantities in the new equilibrium, other things remaining unchanged. So the coefficient of *PCY* in both the reduced-form equations is positive. An increase in the number of auxiliaries would shift the supply curve outward and result in lower prices and a greater quantity of services in equilibrium. Hence, the coefficient of *AX* is negative in equation (5) and positive in equation (6). The net result of a specified shift in both demand and supply on equilibrium prices and quantities can only be determined by evaluating each equation for the different values of the variables concerned.

To determine the equilibrium values of *P* and *Q* with a dental insurance program in effect, we may proceed as follows. The price elasticity of demand evaluated at the equilibrium values of $15.62 and 4,476 sittings equals −1.56. The percentage increase in the number of sittings demanded under a 20 percent copayment plan would be (1.56) × (80) = 125 percent. If we know the percentage increase in the number of sittings demanded (that is, 125 percent), we may use the estimated demand curve to determine by how much incomes would have had to rise to produce the same 125 percent increase in sittings. Assuming other things constant, the equivalent income rise may readily be determined.

Consider equation (3), rewritten as equation (7) below:

$$Q = 6596 - 446P + 1.64PCY - 36FL \quad (7)$$

The new *Q*, call it *Q′*, would be such that:

$$Q' - \overline{Q} = 1.64\,(PCY' - PCY) = 1.25\overline{Q} \quad (8)$$

where *PCY′* is the unknown new income level. Therefore,

$$(PCY' - PCY) = \frac{1.25\overline{Q}}{1.64} \quad (9)$$

where *PCY′* is now the only unknown and may be solved for directly. In this case,

$$\begin{aligned} PCY' = PCY + \frac{1.25\overline{Q}}{1.64} &= 3921 + (.76)\,(4476) \\ &= 3921 + 3402 \quad (10) \\ &= 7323 \end{aligned}$$

Thus, the program has the same effect on the quantity of sittings demanded as a $3,402 increase in per capita incomes to $7,323.

In order to insure the reliability of the model results, the equations naturally were estimated on the subsample consisting of all those dentists who responded to the questionnaire concerning the number of patient sittings, annual income, the number of chairs and assistants, and the number of hours worked. In addition, this subsample comprised only those who responded on all five price questions. Dentists were asked what price they charged for a cleaning, a one-surface amalgam filling, a single extraction, an acrylic jacket crown, and a complete upper acrylic-base denture. Only those who reported a price for each of these procedures were included in the subsample on the assumption that only those who were willing to provide such information would have provided reliable information for the other questions to which they responded.

APPENDIX D: THE IMPACT OF THE REGULATIONS ON THE EARNINGS OF DENTISTS

The impact of the regulations on hourly earnings is estimated in equation (1) below:

$$HOURE = -2.03 + \underset{(2.93)^{***}}{.40EXP} - \underset{(-3.29)^{***}}{.01EXP^2} + \underset{(1.4)^{*}}{.50EDUC} \quad (1)$$

$$- \underset{(-.60)}{.03DNPOP} + \underset{(.32)}{.01PCY} + \underset{(2.05)^{**}}{.07FAIL} + \underset{(1.40)^{*}}{.42EXAUX} - \underset{(-2.56)^{***}}{3.35PVSEM}$$

$$R^2 = .07 \qquad F = 3.55^{***} \qquad N = 420$$

(*t*-statistics are in parentheses)
*significant at the 10 percent level, one-tailed *t*-test
**significant at the 5 percent level, one-tailed *t*-test
***significant at the 1 percent level, one-tailed *t*-test

In this equation, *HOURE* = hourly earnings, *EXP* = years of labor force experience, EXP^2 = the square of *EXP*, *EDUC* = the number of years of education, *DNPOP* = the number of active dentists per 100,000 civilian population in the state, *PCY* = per capita incomes in the state, *FAIL* = the average failure rate on the state license exam for the 1960–1969 decade, *EXAUX* = the expanded-duty dummy, *PVSEM* = 1 if self-employed, 0 if an employee.

NOTES

NOTES TO CHAPTER I

[1] See: U.S. Congress, House of Representatives, Committee on Interstate and Foreign Commerce, *Report on Health Manpower Act of 1974,* 93rd Congress, 2nd session, November 1974, pp. 6-7; U.S. Congress, Senate, Committee on Labor & Public Welfare, *Report on Health Professions Educational Assistance Act of 1974,* 93rd Congress, 2nd session, September 1974, p. 53.

[2] U.S. Congress, House of Representatives, Committee on Interstate and Foreign Commerce, *Hearings on H.R. 4999, 8774, 8833, Summary Statement of the American Dental Association,* 87th Congress, 2nd session, January 1962, p. 178.

[3] Bureau of Health Manpower Education, *Trends in Program Statistics: Grants, Awards and Loans FY 1957-1972* (Washington, D. C.: U.S. Department of Health, Education & Welfare, 1973), p. 6. See also U.S. General Accounting Office, *Congressional Objectives of Federal Loans and Scholarships to Health Professions Students Not Being Met,* Report No. B-164031(2) (Washington, D. C.: May 1974), p. i.

[4] U.S. Congress, House of Representatives, Subcommittee on Public Health and Environment of the Committee on Interstate & Foreign Commerce, *Hearings on National Insurance—Implications,* 93rd Congress, 1st & 2nd sessions, August 1974, p. 206.

[5] Ibid., pp. 207, 214.

[6] John Holahan, *Financing Health Care for the Poor,* (Lexington, Massachusetts: D. C. Heath & Co., 1975), pp. 3, 27.

[7] George M. Gluck, "Dental Services Under Medicaid in Massachusetts," *Journal of Public Health Dentistry,* vol. 31 (Winter 1971), pp. 14-26.

[8] Holahan, *Financing Health Care,* p. 5.

[9] See, for example, J. T. O'Rourke et al., *Dental Education in the United States* (Philadelphia, Pa.: W. B. Saunders Co., 1941) and William McCluggage, *A History of the American Dental Association* (Chicago: American Dental Association, 1959). For a brief summary of some of the historical developments related to the accreditation of dental schools, the development of state examining boards and interstate mobility, see Alex Maurizi, *Economic Essays on the Dental Profession* (Iowa City, Iowa: College of Business Administration, 1969), pp. 48-50. For a valuable summary of some recent developments in regional dental board licensure, see Edward Lusterman, "A Critical Reevaluation of State Boards of Dentistry," *Journal of the American Dental Association,* vol. 84 (January 1972), pp. 103-111.

[10] For a recent discussion of this issue for dentists as well as other health professionals, see U.S. Department of Health, Education and Welfare, *Report on Licensure and Related Health Personnel Credentialing,* June 1971, pp. 1-50; U.S. Department of Health, Education and Welfare, *Developments in Health Manpower Licensure: A Follow-Up to the 1971 Report on Licensure and Related Health Personnel Credentialing,* June 1973; U.S. Department of Health, Education and Welfare, *State Licensing of Health Occupations,* October 1967.

[11] See U.S. Federal Trade Commission, *Regulation of the Television Repair Industry in Louisiana and California* (Washington, D. C., November 1974); Lee Benham, "The Effect of Advertising on the Price of Eyeglasses," *Journal of Law*

and Economics, vol. 15 (October 1972), pp. 337-352; John Cady, *Drugs on the Market* (Lexington, Massachusetts: Lexington Books, 1975).

NOTES TO CHAPTER II

[1] The landmark in the field of human capital inquiry is, of course, Gary Becker, *Human Capital* (New York: National Bureau of Economic Research, 1964). Other empirical works include W. Lee Hansen, "Total and Private Rates of Return to Investment in Schooling," *Journal of Political Economy*, vol. 81 (April 1963), pp. 128-141, and Bruce Wilkinson, "Present Values of Lifetime Earnings for Different Occupations," *Journal of Political Economy*, vol. 74 (December 1966), pp. 556-572.

[2] For a more detailed mathematical formulation of the dental rate of return, see Maurizi, *Economic Essays on the Dental Profession*, pp. 11-37.

[3] See Simon Rottenberg, "On Choice in Labor Markets," *Industrial & Labor Relations Review*, vol. 9 (January 1956), pp. 183-199, for a discussion of the importance of non-monetary factors as well as monetary factors in influencing occupational choice.

[4] Richard Freeman, "Training Lags and the Cobweb Pattern in Engineering," in his *The Market for College-Trained Manpower* (Cambridge, Mass.: Harvard University Press, 1971).

[5] William Mann and Grace Parkin, "The Dental School Applicant," *Journal of Dental Education*, vol. 24 (March 1960), p. 29.

[6] Bureau of Economic Research, *The 1959 Survey of Dental Practice* (Chicago: American Dental Association, 1961), p. 37.

[7] See Maurizi, *Economic Essays on the Dental Profession*, p. 34, for further discussion of this point.

[8] See Milton Friedman, "The Supply of Factors of Production," in his *Price Theory: A Provisional Text* (Chicago: Aldine Publishing Co., 1971), pp. 211-225, and Gary Becker, *Economic Theory* (New York: Alfred Knopf, 1971), pp. 166-176.

[9] Frank Sloan recently studied applicants to medical school and demonstrated that they are influenced by such determinants of the rate of return as tuition, physician's income and income foregone. See Frank Sloan, "The Demand for Higher Education: The Case of Medical School Applicants," *Journal of Human Resources*, vol. 6 (Fall 1971), pp. 466-489. Sloan also calculated rates of return to physicians for three different years in another study. See Frank Sloan, "Lifetime Earnings and Physicians Choice of Specialty," *Industrial and Labor Relations Review*, vol. 24 (October 1970), pp. 47-56. This series of rates of return is too short compared to that available for dentistry to be of much assistance.

[10] D. G. Fish and B. I. Brown, "A Comparison of Applicants and Applications to Canadian Medical and Dental Schools, 1965-66," *Canadian Medical Association Journal*, vol. 95 (July 9, 1966), p. 70.

[11] Mann and Parkin, "The Dental School Applicant," p. 29.

[12] Council on Dental Education, *Dental Student Register* and *Annual Report on Dental Education* (Chicago: American Dental Association); the former was published annually until 1967, the latter has been published annually since 1967.

[13] See, for example, Council on Dental Education, *Annual Report: 1971/72*, p. 5.

[14] Mann and Parkin, "The Dental School Applicant," p. 17.

[15] Bureau of Health Manpower Education, *Trends in Program Statistics*, p. 67.

[16] U.S. General Accounting Office, *Congressional Objectives*, pp. 7-24.

[17] Ibid., pp. 24-27.

[18] Ibid., p. 7.

[19] Ibid., p. 7.

[20] Ibid., p. 11.

[21] Ibid., p. 14.

[22] Ibid., p. 14.
[23] Ibid., p. 12.
[24] Ibid., p. 12.
[25] Ibid., p. 12.
[26] Ibid., p. 12.
[27] Ibid., p. 13.
[28] Ibid., p. 13.
[29] Ibid., p. 14.
[30] Ibid., p. 8.
[31] Ibid., p. 9.
[32] Ibid., p. 9.
[33] Ibid., p. 9.
[34] Ibid., p. 9.
[35] Ibid., p. 21.
[36] Ibid., p. 21.
[37] Ibid., p. 25.
[38] Ibid., p. 25.
[39] Ibid., p. 24.
[40] Paul J. Feldstein, *Financing Dental Care: An Economic Analysis* (Lexington, Mass.: Lexington Books, 1973), p. 92.
[41] Bureau of Health Manpower, *Trends in Program Statistics*, p. 14.

NOTES TO CHAPTER III

[1] Paul Feldstein has also developed a simple model for much the same purpose. The two models differ in several ways, however. First, our model is estimated from the 1962 American Dental Association *Survey of Dental Practice*, using data from individual dental practices. Feldstein was limited to regional summary data from several different years. Second, the models differ in the variables specifying the demand and supply equations. Fluoride is added on the demand side in our model and the number of chairs, assistants, and hours worked by the dentist are used on the supply side in our model. Moreover, in our model, the endogenous variable measuring quantity is the number of annual patient visits to the dentist. In Feldstein's model, this is put on a per capita basis as are all of his other variables. Finally, our model attempts to estimate the impact of a dental insurance program on equilibrium prices and quantities. Feldstein, on the other hand, specifies the effect on quantities assuming various equilibrium prices and demand price elasticities. Despite these significant differences, however, there is some similarity in the estimates of total expenditures and federal expenditures in the two models. See Feldstein, *Financing Dental Care*, pp. 201-203.

[2] See John Sicomi, "Prevention and Control of Periodontal Disease," *Journal of the American Dental Association*, vol. 83 (December 1971), pp. 1271-1287; Bruce Douglas, Donald Wallace, Monroe Lerner, and Sylvia Coppersmith, "Impact of Water Fluoridation on Dental Practice and Dental Manpower," *Journal of the American Dental Association*, vol. 84 (February 1972), pp. 355-370; John Stolpe, Robert Mecklenburg, and Robert Lathrop, "The Effectiveness of an Educational Program on Oral Health in Schools for Improving the Application of Knowledge," *Journal of Public Health Dentistry*, vol. 31 (Winter 1971), pp. 48-59, for a discussion of a number of factors affecting the demand for dental services. The inadequacy of data on many of these factors makes it necessary to concentrate on a few factors in order to develop a model of the national dental care market.

[3] For a discussion of the effects of fluoridation in conjunction with the impact of consumer incomes on the demand for dental services, see Charles Upton and William Silverman, "The Demand for Dental Services," *Journal of Human Resources*, vol. 7 (Spring 1972), pp. 250-261.

[4] The supply side discussion closely resembles that relating to the production function for dental services constructed earlier. See Maurizi, *Economic Essays on the Dental Profession,* pp. 57-70.

[5] Ibid., p. 68.

[6] Byron Hollinshead, *The Survey of Dentistry* (Washington, D. C.: The American Council on Education, 1961), p. 478.

[7] Moreover, it should be noted that there are differences in the output of the dental firm according to what kind of auxiliaries are employed. The increase in output from adding a hygienist or assistant is significantly greater than that from adding a secretary/receptionist. For simplicity, however, we assume that any one kind of full-time assistant is equivalent to any other. See Maurizi, *Economic Essays on the Dental Profession,* p. 58, for a more detailed discussion on this point.

[8] Feldstein, *Financing Dental Care,* p. 144.

[9] Ron Anderson and Lee Benham, "Factors Affecting the Relationship Between Family Income and Medical Care Consumption," in Herb Klarman, ed., *Empirical Studies in Health Economics* (Baltimore: Johns Hopkins Press, 1970), p. 86.

[10] Upton and Silverman, "The Demand for Dental Services," p. 250.

[11] Feldstein, *Financing Dental Care,* p. 144.

[12] Ibid.

[13] For a discussion of a simple simultaneous equation model and its associated reduced form, see Alpha Chiang, *Fundamental Methods of Mathematical Economics* (New York: McGraw-Hill, 1967), pp. 185-189.

[14] For 1970 values of K, AX and HRS, see Bureau of Economic Research, American Dental Association, *The 1971 Survey of Dental Practice* (Chicago: American Dental Association, 1972), pp. 17, 26, 30-32, respectively. For 1970 values of PCY, see U.S. Census Bureau, *Statistical Abstract of the United States: 1973* (Washington, D. C.: U.S. Government Printing Office, 1974), p. 380; for the 1969 value of FL, see U.S. Department of Health, Education and Welfare, *Annual Fluoridation Census: 1969* (Washington, D. C.: Public Health Service, 1970), p. 9. The value of FL reported is as of December 31, 1969. The 1970 mean values used for K, AX, HRS, PCY and FL are 2.4, 1.56, 1987, 3921 and 43.0, respectively.

[15] U.S. Department of Health, Education and Welfare, *Health Resource Statistics* (Washington, D. C.: U.S. Department of Health, Education and Welfare, 1970).

[16] For several examples of how these features might be designed in combination, see Feldstein, *Financing Dental Care,* p. 144.

[17] It should be noted that the demand-price elasticity must be reevaluated at the new point of equilibrium in order to determine the effects of an insurance program in this and in the subsequent two examples.

NOTES TO CHAPTER IV

[1] O'Rourke, *Dental Education in the United States,* p. 267.

[2] McCluggage, *History of the American Dental Association,* p. 385.

[3] Milton Friedman, "Occupational Licensure," in his *Capitalism and Freedom* (Chicago: University of Chicago Press, 1963), pp. 137-160. See also Alex Maurizi, "Occupational Licensing and the Public Interest," *Journal of Political Economy,* vol. 82 (March/April 1974), pp. 399-413.

[4] Bureau of Economic Research, American Dental Association, *Facts About States for the Dentist Seeking a Location* (Chicago: American Dental Association, 1973), pp. 11-12.

[5] Ibid., p. 13.

[6] Ibid., pp. 13, 19.

[7] Ibid., pp. 11-12. For an excellent discussion of the restrictive licensing of dental auxiliaries, see Owen MacBride, "Restrictive Licensing of Dental Paraprofessionals," *Yale Law Journal,* vol. 83 (March 1974), pp. 806-826.

[8] Advertising, especially price advertising, is generally regarded as unethical conduct and is consequently prohibited. For example, unprofessional conduct in California is defined to include "the advertising of definite or fixed prices for professional services," "the advertising of any free dental work or free examination," and "the advertising to guarantee any dental service, or to perform any dental operation painlessly." Of course, unprofessional conduct is a basis for suspension or revocation of a dentist's license. See Board of Dental Examiners, *Dental Practice Act,* Consumers Affairs Department, Sacramento, California, p. 20.

[9] U.S. Bureau of the Census, *Public Use Samples of Basic Records from the 1970 Census: Description and Technical Documentation* (Washington, D. C.: U.S. Government Printing Office, 1972), pp. 191-193.

[10] The available evidence indicates that those who pass the license exam are more likely to have attended a dental school in the state or have a previous residence in the state than those who do not pass. See Hollinshead, *The Survey of Dentistry,* p. 391, and Coordinating Council for Higher Education, *Dental Education and Manpower* (Sacramento, California: California Office of State Printing, 1964), p. 10.

[11] See Maurizi, "Occupational Licensing and the Public Interest," for a discussion and empirical test of the proposition that the licensure failure rate for an occupation is affected by the extent of excess demand for the services of members of that occupation.

[12] The data was obtained from Council on Dental Education, American Dental Association, *Requirements and Registration Data: State Dental Examining Boards* (Chicago: American Dental Association, 1961, 1962, 1963, 1965, 1968); Bureau of Economic Research, American Dental Association, *Facts About States,* 1969, 1970, 1971; and from the Council on Dental Education directly.

[13] See Owen MacBride, "Restrictive Licensing of Dental Paraprofessionals," p. 813, for a more detailed discussion of the developments since 1967. The source of the data used in the analysis for the year 1969 is Donald Johnson and Stuart Bernstein, "Classification of States Regarding Expanding Duties for Dental Auxiliaries and Selected Aspects of Dental Licensure—1970," *American Journal of Public Health,* vol. 62 (February 1972), pp. 208-215. More recent investigations of this subject include: Council on Dental Education, "Expanded Functions Delegated to Dental Hygienists and Dental Assistants," *American Dental Association* January 1974, unpublished paper; D. W. Johnson and F. M. Holz, *Legal Provisions on Expanded Functions for Dental Hygienists and Dental Assistants* (Washington, D. C.: U.S. Department of Health, Education and Welfare, 1974).

[14] Becker, *Human Capital,* pp. 7-36.

[15] For a recent discussion of the relation between education and earnings after adjusting for ability differences, see Burton Weisbrod and Peter Karpoff, "Monetary Returns to College Education, Student Ability and College Quality," *Review of Economics and Statistics,* vol. 50 (November 1968), pp. 491-497.

[16] Self-employed dentists are found in both incorporated and unincorporated businesses. In either case, we define earnings to be the summation of wage earnings and earnings from independent professional practice, since the dentist may pay himself a wage. Those in incorporated businesses receive their earnings both as wages and salaries and also as a return to their investment which is sometimes reported as "other" income. Those in unincorporated enterprises report all earnings from the business as earnings from independent professional practice. There is therefore some underestimation of earnings for the incorporated self-employed dentist in our definition of earnings. Since 96 percent of self-employed dentists are found in unincorporated businesses, however, the effect of this bias is likely to be small.

[17] See MacBride, "Restrictive Practices of Dental Paraprofessionals," pp. 815-816.

[18] See Ibid., pp. 809-810, for a comprehensive list of the studies that have been made of the effects of using expanded-duty personnel under controlled experimental conditions—effects both on the productivity of the dental firm and on the quality of care administered by the expanded-duty personnel as compared to the quality of the same care administered by the dentist.

[19] Ibid., pp. 817-825.

[20] For further discussion in this connection, see Benjamin Shimberg, Barbara Esser and Daniel Kruger, *Occupational Licensing: Practices and Policies* (Washington, D. C.: Public Affairs Press, 1973), pp. 240-249.

NOTES TO CHAPTER V

[1] Concern over the existence of externalities emerges because an equilibrium position for an economy may not be Pareto-optimal when externalities exist. Externalities are generally the result of some economic activities having inappropriate prices or no prices at all. See E. J. Mishan, *Cost-Benefit Analysis* (New York: Praeger Publications, 1971), pp. 101-104; Becker, *Economic Theory*, pp. 84-89; Milton Friedman, "The Role of Government in a Free Society," in his *Capitalism and Freedom*, pp. 22-36.

[2] For a benefit-cost analysis of the polio prevention program, see Burton Weisbrod, "Costs and Benefits of Medical Research: A Case Study of Poliomyelitis," *Journal of Political Economy*, vol. 79 (May/June 1971), pp. 527-544. For related discussions, see Weisbrod, *Economics of Public Health: Measuring the Economics of Diseases* (Philadelphia: University of Pennsylvania Press, 1961), and Robin Barlow, "The Economic Effects of Malaria Eradication," *American Economic Review*, vol. 57 (May 1967), pp. 130-148.

[3] See Richard Coffman, "The Economics of Fluoridation," unpublished paper, December 1973. This paper was based on the author's "The Economics of Fluoridation" (Unpublished Ph.D. dissertation, University of Washington, 1972).

[4] See, for example, the litigation surrounding the patents by the Wright brothers on the invention of the airplane, discussed in Fred Kelly, *The Wright Brothers* (New York: Ballantine Books, 1969), pp. 176-183. Even though they won all their patent suits in America and in Europe, the cost was considerable. Moreover, the fact that they won did not assure their collection of royalties for the use of their patented inventions. Dentistry has its own history of patent controversy concerning the use of amalgam as a filling material. See Robert W. McCluggage, *A History of the American Dental Association*, pp. 67-87, 204-206.

[5] See Tibor Scitovsky, *Welfare and Competition* (Chicago: Richard Irwin, 1959), pp. 335-336.

[6] Armen A. Alchian and William R. Allen, *University Economics*, second edition (Belmont, California: Wadsworth Publishing Co., 1968), pp. 217-218.

[7] Milton Friedman, "The Role of Government in Education," in his *Capitalism and Freedom*, pp. 100-107.

[8] See, for example, Alchian and Allen, *University Economics*, pp. 70-71.

[9] Friedman, "Occupational Licensure," p. 148.

[10] See Feldstein, *Financing Dental Care*, pp. 40-42.

[11] Mishan, *Cost-Benefit Analysis*, pp. 105-108.

[12] Holahan, *Financing Health Care*, pp. 23-26.

[13] U.S. Congress, House, Subcommittee on Public Health and Environment, *Hearings on National Health Insurance*, p. 207.

[14] Robert Strauss and Colin Cornett, "Locational Aspects of Welfare Participation in North Carolina," University of North Carolina, 1975, unpublished paper.

[15] See Feldstein, *Financing Dental Care*, pp. 175-189, for a similar discussion.

NOTES TO APPENDIX A

[1] U.S. Congress, Senate, Committee on Labor and Public Welfare, *Health Professions Act*, p. 10.

[2] Ibid., p. 11.

[3] Ibid., pp. 12-13.

[4] Ibid., pp. 13-14.

[5] U.S. Congress, House, Committee on Interstate and Foreign Commerce, *Health Manpower Act*, pp. 2, 135-151.

[6] U.S. Congress, Senate, Committee on Labor and Public Welfare, *Health Professions Act*, pp. 12-13.

[7] U.S. General Accounting Office, *Congressional Objectives*, pp. 4-5.

[8] Ibid., p. 6.

[9] U.S. Congress, Senate, Committee on Labor and Public Welfare, *Health Professions Act*, pp. 15-16.

[10] U.S. Congress, House, Committee on Interstate and Foreign Commerce, *Health Manpower Act*, pp. 125, 130.

[11] U.S. Congress, Senate, Committee on Labor and Public Welfare, *Health Professions Act*, pp. 5-7.

[12] U.S. Congress, House, Committee on Interstate and Foreign Commerce, *Health Manpower Act*, pp. 2-3.

[13] Ibid.

NOTES TO APPENDIX C

[1] Present theoretical knowledge of two-stage estimators is limited to their asymptotic properties, particularly the asymptotic variance. For this reason, standard errors are generally reported below the two-stage estimates. See, for example, Ronald J. Wonnacott and Thomas H. Wonnacott, *Econometrics* (New York: John Wiley and Sons, 1970), p. 398.

	DATE DUE		
MY 27 '94			